THE 30-DAY
NATURAL
HORMONE
PLAN

THE 30-DAY
NATURAL
HORMONE
PLAN

Look and Feel Young Again–
Without Synthetic HRT

ERIKA SCHWARTZ, M.D.

WARNER BOOKS

An AOL Time Warner Company

Warner Books, Inc., 1271 Avenue of the Americas, New York, NY 10020

Visit our Web site at www.twbookmark.com.

An AOL Time Warner Company

Printed in the United States of America
First Printing: January 2004
10 9 8 7 6 5 4 3 2 1

The Library of Congress Cataloging-in-Publication Data
Schwartz, Erika.
    The 30-day natural hormone plan : look and feel young again without synthetic HRT / Erika Schwartz.
        p. cm.
Includes bibliographical references and index.
    ISBN 0-446-53255-X
        1. Hormones—Health aspects. 2. Dietary supplements. 3. Hormone therapy—Popular works. 4. Middle aged women—Health and hygiene. I. Title: Thirty day natural hormone plan. II. Title.
QP571.S39 2004
613'.04244—dc22   2003015188

Book design by Giorgetta B. McRee

To my family

Acknowledgments

As I finish my third book, I realize more than ever that the number of people I have come to rely on is rapidly expanding. While their positions in my life may change, their cumulative importance grows. Longtime collaborators and peers are now friends, while others, more recent additions, have brought new help to my mission to provide valid, clear, logical information and solutions to my patients and readers. All have one thing in common: They believe in me and in my message.

To them and to you my readers, I promise to be worthy of your trust and continue my quest to improve health care by speaking the truth with kindness and respect toward every human being.

While my thanks are going to all my patients and supporters, there are a few people I must single out for their particularly significant input into the making of *The 30-Day Natural Hormone Plan*.

Deborah Schneider, my agent and friend, thank you for never letting me down. Every new book I write is a testimonial to your encouragement and persistence. Like Ace and Gracie, we will survive.

Sharyn Kolberg, you came into my life at the best possible moment and made it even better with your brilliant mind, your beautiful writing, and your consistency. Thank you.

Peter Karamanlakis, my colleague and shiny new M.D. Your commitment and unbridled enthusiasm are guarantees you will make the medical profession proud of you. I am.

Laurence Kirshbaum, president of Warner Books, and Diana Baroni, executive editor, thank you for publishing my books and adding the much-needed personal touch in a tough industry.

Laura Jorstad, my copyeditor, thank you for your kind words.

Maria Levada, M.D., from college until now, thirty years later, you are still kind, loving, and a great doctor and friend.

Spencer Falk, thank you for making it easy for me to take the spotlight and never letting me go too far into the dumps just because the sun isn't always shining.

Odette Fodor, Costel Cristache, Patrick Kerr, Joe Bova, Dan and Wendy Cooper, Marty and Geri Singerman, Damon and Caroline Tragni, my friends and coworkers, I thank you.

Last and most important, Ken, Lisa, Katie, Bethany, Ben, Katie C., and Nick, the only thing that matters in life is a kind, honest, loving family. Thank you for being mine.

Contents

Preface

In July 2002, I suddenly found myself swamped with phone calls, e-mails, and lecture requests from consumer outlets and medical establishments. They all wanted to know about natural hormones.

At the time, I was making the rounds at bookstores, on television, and on radio promoting my previous book *The Hormone Solution*, which explained the use of natural forms of hormone replacement to treat myriad problems caused by hormone imbalances. That book is really a primer on the physiology and role of hormones—what they are and what they do. It's important information that every woman (and man, too) should know. I had become accustomed to speaking about hormones in this light.

But one day in July I realized I had to do something different.

For starters, women had been telling me since the book came out that they wanted specific information about what to do on a daily basis to maintain their hormone health. I realized that I had to talk about hormones in a way that everyone could understand and use without feeling obligated to become an expert in endocrinology. I needed to eliminate the medical lingo, the source of the all-too-large distance between the public and medical information.

And then there was the NIH bombshell.

Just a few days earlier, the National Institutes of Health had abruptly halted a ten-year study (called the Women's Health Initiative) on synthetic hormones. The study was less than half complete, yet the risks to the women taking part in it were too great to continue. Now millions of women who were taking these same hormones at the recommendation of their physicians were left wondering: *How dangerous are these hormones? Are they bad for all women? Are all hormones the same? Are there any safe and realistic options?*

Now was not the time for a lecture on the physiology of hormones. I wanted my audience to feel better and less scared.

I took a deep breath and, hoping my own hormones would stay
in balance for the following forty-five minutes, began a talk I was
to give hundreds of times in the coming months to women and
their doctors.

It outlined the thirty-day program that my patients and I had
been following for five years—a plan that the public and medical
profession are now fascinated with. I talked about how the program
provides a lasting and safe solution to problems of hormone imbalance regardless of age. It includes supervised use of natural hormones, supplements, vitamins, diet, exercise, and lifestyle. And it
has been successful for maintaining health and a youthful appearance in thousands of patients.

The work I speak about is in the book you are about to read. It is
the total package that will bring balance and health into the rest of
your life.

Introduction: Why the 30-Day Plan?

Recently, a patient of mine in her midfifties came to see me. She was a few weeks away from heart bypass surgery and wanted to know what she could do to make her recovery as easy and complication-free as possible. I gave her some options and some suggestions to enhance the healing process.

She interrupted me and said, "I don't want options and suggestions. I want you to tell me exactly what I need to do—otherwise I won't do it."

So we sat down and drew up a specific, delineated plan for her to follow.

I understood her request; I hear it often from my women patients who are dealing with their bodies' confusing and anxiety-inducing changes. Their plea is very simple: "Tell me what to do." That's why I wrote this book. In it, I will tell you, specifically, what you need to do for thirty days in order to jump-start (and then maintain) a healthy rest-of-your-life.

Not everyone, I know, wants or needs to be given exact instructions. Thus, I've also given you options so that if you don't like a specific meal or a particular exercise I recommend, you can substitute other choices that better fit your taste or lifestyle. Whatever way you choose to follow the plan, you'll find yourself feeling healthier and more energized, and looking younger in the bargain.

WHAT WILL THE PLAN DO FOR YOU?

This is the only program that integrates every aspect of your life to prevent chronic illness and keep you feeling and looking young. The program should be used when you are healthy or when you are sick; it should become your mantra for the twenty-first century. Start the program today. It provides simple ways to:

- Eat right.
- Integrate exercise in your life.
- Help you find time to get enough rest.
- Identify essential basic and necessary supplements and vitamins.
- Access natural hormones you need to create your proper hormone balance.
- Solve many health problems that have been plaguing you since early adulthood.

We are all looking for solutions, and that's what this program is all about.

The 30-Day Plan will help you:

- Identify the existence of a problem by learning how significant changes in your own life impact you directly.
- Identify the specific symptoms in your physiologic or mental state brought on by hormone changes.
- Connect hormone changes to symptoms.
- Solve specific problems by following the 30-Day Plan and integrating all the pieces of your life into the program.
- Individualize the application of the steps to enhance your life.

WHAT IS THE PLAN? DIET, EXERCISE, VITAMINS, SUPPLEMENTS, AND NATURAL HORMONES

I purposely made this a simple plan. If you're like most of my patients, you don't have the time to analyze the contents of your food or follow complicated and rigid diets that add stress to your life. Nor do you always have the time to follow a lengthy exercise program, so I have created an integrated exercise regimen that fits everyone's lifestyle. You probably know that you need to take vitamins and supplements—but the information that bombards us daily in this area can be truly daunting. That's why I created a combination of vitamins and supplements that will help you balance your hormones without overwhelming you with too many pills or too much expense. And last but certainly not least, I recommend a program of natural hormone supplementation to get your body back in balance and to reduce or eliminate specific problems caused by hormones out of whack.

THE MANY PARTS THAT MAKE UP THE WHOLE

As much as we have tried to find the magic pill that will cure everything and keep us young and beautiful forever, we know it doesn't exist. No real program to balance your hormones and keep you young and fit can be limited to one vitamin, or one supplement, or even one lifestyle change. The cure-all is found in the integration of our lives. Just as we know the puzzle of our lives is made of hundreds, if not thousands, of pieces, there are many parts that help the 30-Day Plan balance our hormones, integrate our lives, and return us to our younger, fitter selves.

Each part is easy to follow and opens the door to the next one. The domino effect you will experience is natural and logical. Just by following the simple progression in the next few chapters, the results will amaze you:

- Start by identifying your problem areas.
- Get a thorough medical checkup to make sure you have no underlying medical problems that need treatment.
- Discuss the 30-Day Plan with your doctor and have him or her help you implement the steps.
- Take your vitamins and supplements as advised in the program.
- Balance your body with natural hormones as advised in the program.
- Start the journal and use it faithfully.
- Start the diet and follow guidelines or specific instructions. Do what works best for you. If you aren't sure what works, try both ways.
- Start and follow the exercise and activities program and stay with it.
- Address the lifestyle issues progressively as soon as you identify them.
- Take total control and responsibility over your physical and mental life.
- Integrate all the parts and watch your life improve over thirty days.
- Use the 30-Day Plan as a guideline for a healthy, long-term way of life.

I came up with the 30-Day Plan when I began to have the signs and symptoms of menopause that were making my own life miserable. When I saw how much it helped me, I began recommending that my patients follow the same path. Now hundreds of women have used the plan to balance their hormones and greatly improve their lives. Read this book and see how easy it can be to make a change for a better, healthier life.

Author's Note

The program described in this book is not intended to be a substitute for medical care and advice. You are advised to consult with your health care professional with regard to all matters relating to your health, including matters that may require diagnosis or medical attention. In particular, if you have any special condition requiring medical attention, or if you are taking or have been advised to take (or to refrain from taking) any medication, you should consult regularly with your physician.

The identity of some of the patients referred to in this book, and certain details about them, have been modified or are presented in composite form.

The information provided in this book is based on sources that the author believes to be reliable, and information regarding products and companies is current as of August 2003.

PART I

HORMONES 101

1

◯

What Everyone Needs to Know

Hormones are powerful agents of change in our body. They cause direct changes in our bodily functions and facilitate our body's reactions to environmental changes. All of us—men, women, adults, and adolescents—experience constant hormone fluctuations. How we look and feel is the direct result of our hormone balance.

When our hormones are in balance, meaning *all* our hormones are working together well, the results are amazing. Our skin looks radiant and fresh, our minds work smoothly, we remember things, we focus well, our weight and moods are stable, our sex drive soars. We are young and healthy.

When our hormones are out of balance, problems can develop. We have difficulty focusing, we get tired and stay tired, we can't catch up on sleep. We become insomniacs, lose interest in sex, get bloated, and gain weight. We develop aches and pains in our joints; our skin gets wrinkled and dry; we get heart disease, digestive problems, arthritis, osteoporosis. We age.

The aging process is the result of years of wear and tear on our body. It mirrors the state of our hormone balance, our genetics, and the type of life we lead.

Understanding how our hormone balance affects everything we do in our lives is key to maintaining health and preventing aging from robbing us of vitality.

The need to understand and make the connection between hormone balance and lifestyle, diet, exercise, stress, sleep, and every part of our lives prompted me to develop the 30-Day Plan.

The goal of the program is to help keep you healthy and youthful for as long as possible. To take you there, we must first gain insight into the connection between health (*hormones in balance*) and physical and mental deterioration (*hormones out of balance*). Once this insight is achieved, the 30-Day Plan helps integrate natural hormones, supplements, diet, exercise, and lifestyle into your whole life and effectively accomplish the dream of staying well and delaying the destructive effects of aging on the body and mind.

This book contains all the simple tools and information you need to accomplish the anti-aging goal and to understand the messages that your own body sends you. In addition to the diet, exercise, and lifestyle portions, I will reinforce the balancing program with simple and easily available combinations of natural hormones and supplements.

The natural hormones I endorse and advise you to use are approved by the U.S. Food and Drug Administration (FDA) and have been on the market for twenty years with long track records of safety along with extensive clinical experience in the United States, Canada, and Europe.

The supplements and vitamins I recommend are backed up by reliable and respected scientific research and substantial clinical data that support their safety and efficacy. They are accepted and in use by both conventional medicine and alternative therapies.

But until now, these products have not been combined in the context of a comprehensive program. My 30-Day Plan is the result of more than twenty-five years of experience as a doctor helping solve all types of hormone problems from which my patients have been suffering. Up to now, the information contained in this book was only available to the limited number of people who could be my patients. Now you and your physician can share the 30-Day Plan and help achieve perfect hormonal balance for your body and mind.

The 30-Day Plan will help you integrate your diet, exercise, and lifestyle into a successful hormone-balancing, anti-aging package that uses common sense and proven medical knowledge.

UNDERSTANDING HORMONES

Before we get started, we need to understand what hormones are, and that they are *all* involved in achieving the balance we need to feel healthy.

Hormones are products of living cells that circulate in our bodily fluids and produce specific effects on the activity of other cells far removed from the organs where the hormones are made. They stimulate or inhibit the actions of cells everywhere in the body. No organ is left untouched by the actions of hormones.

There are hundreds of hormones in our bodies, and they have innumerable jobs. They regulate all bodily functions and interact with each other at all times. No hormone acts on its own. The action of one hormone affects the action of many others and the results vary, depending on infinite internal and external factors.

Hormones are produced through chemical processes by glands and organs in specialized cells. They are made from fatty acids, various combinations of protein components called amino acids, and certain sugar molecules. Most hormones are, in fact, derived from a familiar substance, cholesterol. This is one reason cholesterol should not be dismissed as no more than the culprit behind fatty deposits in our arteries that cause heart disease or stroke. Without cholesterol, our body cannot make hormones—and that's an even graver danger.

Here's a partial list of the better-known and -researched hormones. This list will give you an idea of their names and how their presence is ubiquitous:

- Insulin.
- Growth hormone.
- Thyroid hormones (triiodothyonine [T_3] and thyroxine [T_4]).
- Parathyroid hormone (parathormone).
- Calcitonin.
- Estrogen.
- Progesterone.
- Testosterone.
- Stomach hormones (gastrin, pepsin, trypsin, secretin, and others).

- Pancreatic hormones (insulin, glucagon).
- Adrenal hormones (cortisol, aldosterone).
- Kidney hormones (renin).
- Lung hormones (angiotensin).
- Brain hormones (serotonin, melatonin, dopamine, luteinizing hormone, follicle-stimulating hormone, prolactin, adrenaline, endorphins, norepinephrine).

Looking at this list, you probably recognize some familiar names. Some of these, like adrenaline, serotonin, and dopamine, are often called neurotransmitters. They're still hormones, only they're categorized under a specific grouping of hormones that enhance or delay transmission of messages in the nervous system, and in the brain in particular. Another group, estrogen, progesterone, and testosterone, are the sex hormones. Both men and women have all three of them, but they vary in concentration according to your gender.

Some of these hormones are "good" hormones, while others are not. The good hormones help improve well-being and memory, maintain sugar balance, and stimulate positive reactions in your body. The "bad" hormones, when they are out of balance, can be destructive and increase wear and tear on your mind and your internal organs.

Examples of good hormones are: serotonin, progesterone, testosterone, glucagon, aldosterone, dopamine, and growth hormone.

Examples of bad hormones are: cortisol, insulin, and sometimes estrogen.

What's important to remember is that there is no such thing as an independent hormone action. Every action affects everything else going on. Every hormone interacts with others. For us to feel good and stay healthy, every hormone has to work in balance and synchrony. When we look at a list of effects of individual hormones, we are looking at only a small part of the picture.

HORMONES IN BALANCE

If hormones can be said to have a goal in life, it is to maintain what is called homeostasis, which means that they are constantly working to keep us in a state of equilibrium. They strive to maintain balance inside the body regardless of outside environmental conditions. In order to maintain this balance, they react to everything we do. And I mean *everything*—like eating, sleeping, reading, running, breathing, hugging, having sex, daydreaming, sitting, standing, even thinking.

Remember: Many hormones are working at the same time. This is why no one hormone—or no one *anything* (vitamin, food, supplement, medication)—will balance us, keep us young, or protect us from our own individual ways of destroying our bodies.

And this is why your goal in life should be the same as your hormones'—to achieve homeostasis, through which you can stay healthy and enjoy life.

HORMONES OUT OF WHACK

In an ideal world, we'd all be in homeostasis all the time. But even in the best of times, we don't live in an ideal world. We live busy lives, sad lives, happy lives, working lives, playing lives—all at the same time. Our hormones are constantly adapting to the changes we experience throughout every single day.

Remember: Hormone levels change whenever we change. Regardless of age, as long as we are alive, our hormone levels are changing continuously. When our lives take a new direction, when a stress appears or disappears, our hormone balance changes. If we are lucky enough to have a well-balanced life and are aware of these changes, we can preempt or minimize the problems. But even if we're able to rapidly rebalance, we never totally prevent the most common reaction, hormones out of whack.

Lucy was fifty-eight when I first saw her. She had been a physi-cal education teacher. Diet, exercise, and great personal care were part of her life. Two years earlier, she and her husband won the lottery. They didn't have children or family ties in New York where they lived and decided to retire to Florida. With no wor-ries about work or money, they had only sunny days to look for-ward to—until the unexpected happened.

Lucy had sailed through menopause at forty-five with almost no symptoms. But now she suddenly started having severe hot flashes, night sweats, insomnia, and mood swings. Suffering with almost incapacitating symptoms, Lucy was convinced she had cancer. She saw three doctors: an internist, an endocrinologist, and a gynecologist. Diagnoses of Lyme disease, arthritis, dia-betes, thyroid problems, and cancer were considered but dis-carded. Finally one of the physicians told Lucy that her problems were probably hormone related, but there was nothing that could be done.

The physician was right about the cause of her symptoms— her problems *were* an outgrowth of hormone imbalance. But he was wrong when he said there was no solution. When Lucy came to me, I treated her with a combination of natural hor-mones: estradiol and micronized progesterone in cream form. But treating the symptoms is not always enough. I knew it was essential to find out what had triggered Lucy's sudden hormone imbalance.

I asked Lucy to start a journal (see chapter 8). It turned out that for her (as for many other people), retirement was more stressful than her busy life had been. She missed the city life. The stress of the move, and the change of climate and emo-tional environment, had pushed her delicate hormone balance over the edge. Her hormones were going crazy trying to adjust to so many changes at once.

Within three months, following my program of natural hormones, supplementation, and journaling, Lucy gained a better understanding of her new life and began to feel herself again.

Hormones out of whack can be caused by the smallest of changes in your internal and/or external environments. Never underestimate or overlook any part of your life when doing the detective work of finding what caused your hormones to lose their balance.

Unfortunately, it's all too easy to throw your own hormones out of whack. I know; I've done it myself. I have personally been using natural/bioidentical hormones, the supplement regimen, and the 30-Day Plan for more than five years. Occasionally, however, I behave like every other human being and lose my balance. A perfect example: I had been doing well for months. My hormones were in perfect synchrony. My eating habits were impeccable, and my life was running smoothly without too much stress. A perfect time to throw off my hormone balance—and it all started with a cup of coffee.

I love coffee. Unfortunately, coffee doesn't like me, so I generally avoid it. But one day, I found myself with a yen for coffee. I decided to have just one espresso. I did. No symptoms. I advanced to a double. Still no problem. Within three days, I was drinking two cups of coffee a day. I started getting a little heartburn. I took some Zantac. The heartburn was gone and I continued my coffees. I knew the coffee was causing the heartburn, but I chose to ignore that fact.

Within one week, I started waking up in the middle of the night with night sweats. During the day I experienced an occasional hot flash. Within another few days, I found myself exhausted all the time. Soon after, I started craving sweets, and my commitment to exercise suddenly disappeared. Faced with all these changes, I thought I might be taking too high a dose of natural hormones, so I decreased my dose. My symptoms worsened. Finally, after two weeks of feeling crummy, I decided to face reality. My hormones were out of whack and everything I did added to the problem.

I stopped the coffee, went back on my usual dosage of natural hormones, cleaned up my eating act, and got back on track. It took two weeks to get back to normal. The lesson learned? I'm fifty-two, my body cannot tolerate coffee, and I have to listen to it if I want to feel good. The lesson relearned? The balance of hormones is precarious, and one small thing can set off a domino effect, pushing everything out of control.

The 30-Day Plan will help prevent the dominoes from falling and robbing you of precious wellness time. By following the advice in these pages, you will be able to quickly identify the culprits that disturb your hormone balance. By the time you're finished with this book, your hormones will no longer be a mystery, and understanding how to help maintain their balance will be second nature.

MENARCHE TO MENOPAUSE— WHO SUFFERS FROM HORMONE IMBALANCE?

While preparing to write *The Hormone Solution*, I reviewed the records of five hundred patients (covering the years 1997 through 2001) in my own practice, looking at the age distribution for women with diagnoses related to hormone imbalances. The demographics revealed an almost even distribution between menopausal women and women ranging in age from sixteen to forty-five.

The results seemed unusual, but I was sure I wasn't misdiagnosing these women. They all had thorough and complete medical evaluations and blood tests from other doctors before they came to me. Their extensive and expensive workups confused and scared them, but offered them no solutions. But when I put them on my 30-Day Plan and began balancing their hormones, their symptoms consistently disappeared.

Which led me to ask: *How often do symptoms of hormone imbalance in young women go unnoticed and undiagnosed in the general population?*

Clearly these young women were not aberrations. They were suffering with severe premenstrual syndrome (PMS), bloating, breast tenderness, mood swings, loss of sex drive, hot flashes, and night sweats. These were serious symptoms and needed to be brought into the open and addressed.

I didn't remember reading any medical literature addressing symptoms of hormone imbalance in populations outside the standard menopause age group. Before I put this surprising information into my book, I decided to review the scientific literature and find out what other hormone experts had found.

I turned to the medical literature looking for statistical data on age distribution and frequency of symptoms of hormone imbalance at different ages. Not only did I find nothing on age distribution, but I also found no adequate information on the presence of symptoms of hormone imbalance in other age groups besides menopause.

Medical textbooks of obstetrics and gynecology, internal medicine, and endocrinology, clinical manuals, medical journals in the United States and abroad, rarely addressed the incidence of symptoms of hormone imbalance in young women similar to those suffered by menopausal women. Few, if any, medical textbooks addressed the connection between hormone imbalances and symptoms such as PMS and depression in young women. The only time that medical literature addressed symptoms and connected them to hormone imbalance was when women were either sick or menopausal.

The first people who connected the symptoms of hormone imbalance (PMS, depression, and so forth) to hormone imbalances were doctors who were not writing medical textbooks or journals—they wrote books and articles that were meant to be read by women themselves. Books such as *No More Hot Flashes and Other Good News* by Dr. Penny Wise Budoff (1983), *Women's Bodies, Women's Wisdom: Creating Physical and Emotional Health and Healing* by Dr. Christiane Northrup (first published in 1994), and *Screaming to Be Heard: Hormonal Connections Women Suspect . . . and Doctors Ignore* by Dr. Elizabeth Lee Vliet (1995) asked women to take responsibility for bringing their knowledge to the attention of their physicians.

Over the years, I have found that popular (nonscientific) literature is sometimes ahead of the medical journals because it needs to be in touch with its readers to survive. But in this case, even the nonscientific literature was difficult to find. With the exception of the above-mentioned books, I found few books written before 1996 that specifically addressed symptoms of hormone imbalance in any age group, not even books on menopause (there was one exception—a book written in 1968 by Robert Wilson, called *Feminine*

Forever, which was sponsored by Wyeth [then Ayerst] pharmaceuticals promoting the rejuvenating effects of its new drug Premarin).

Then, in the mid-1990s, the floodgates of menopause burst open. A tide of literature addressing issues surrounding hormone imbalances in menopausal women swept the consumer market. I read every one I could get my hands on. They all addressed menopause and the symptoms created by the loss of hormones associated with aging. But I found myself wondering why anybody would expect the symptoms of hormone imbalance to just appear out of nowhere around the age of forty-five to fifty. Why would we look at hormone changes in a vacuum, as a sudden incident rather than part of the continuum of hormone changes? Isn't life a continuum?

Back in my practice, I continued to see women of all ages with complaints of hormone imbalance. I became determined to acknowledge and validate the presence of the symptoms regardless of age.

The Hormone Solution was published in April 2002. Since then, I've been seeing even more young women in my practice. They call from around the country and around the world, seeking advice and information. Many have been experiencing undiagnosed severe symptoms for years. Others are just fearful of finding themselves out of hormones in their forties and fifties without preparation. They say, "I don't want to wind up like my mother, suddenly old and sick and overwhelmed by symptoms of menopause."

Once you realize that hormone imbalance can occur at any age, you can take a proactive role and learn to identify the symptoms, connect them to hormone issues, and then treat them following a thorough and all-inclusive program. My research enabled me to break down frequency of symptoms according to age into five major groupings. You can use the guidelines for age groupings to help you sift through your own symptoms (but remember—you may experience any of these symptoms at any age).

GROUP 1 (AGES 16–EARLY 20s)

Symptoms

- PMS.
- Bloating.
- Mood swings.
- Acne.

GROUP 2 (AGES MID-20s–MID-30s)

Symptoms

- Bloating.
- Weight gain.
- Postpartum depression.
- PMS.
- Mood swings.
- Fatigue.

GROUP 3 (AGES 30s–EARLY 40s)

Symptoms

- Weight gain.
- Bloating.
- PMS.
- Depression.
- Occasional loss of libido.
- Occasional night sweats.
- Irritability.
- Menstrual irregularity.
- Migraines.
- Fatigue.

GROUP 4 (AGES 45–55)

Symptoms

- Hot flashes.
- Night sweats.
- Insomnia.
- Loss of libido.
- Irritability.
- Mood swings.
- Depression.
- Weight gain.
- Bloating.
- Fatigue.
- Muscle and joint aches.
- Vaginal dryness.

GROUP 5 (AGES 55+)

Symptoms

- Hot flashes.
- Night sweats.
- Fatigue.
- Insomnia.
- Weight gain.
- Loss of libido.
- Arthritis.
- Stiffness in the muscles and joints.
- Chronic constipation.
- Bloating.
- Chronic illnesses (osteoporosis, heart diseases).

LIFE CYCLES AND HORMONES

From puberty to menopause, our bodies constantly manufacture hormones. There is always an ebb and flow of hormonal activity going on, often in cycles. The most familiar of these is the menstrual cycle. There are, however, other equally important cycles that impact our hormone balance, some of them internal and some external.

The internal cycle most readily known and studied is the regular (or irregular) monthly cycle our bodies create to keep hormones in balance and help us perpetuate the species by making young women fertile every month. Menstrual cycles vary during a woman's life span. Menstrual regularity at twenty-eight to thirty days is the norm, but statistical data on frequency and cycling of menstruation show enormous variation. Although we rarely read these facts, it appears that menstruation cycles vary from fifteen to sixty to ninety days in women without any diagnosed illnesses or problems with conception. A growing school of thought affirms that regularity of the menstrual cycle is unimportant as long as fertility is unaffected.

The only problem with unpredictable periods is in the area of pregnancy prevention. Ovulation, and the forty-eight hours of fertility that ensue, occurs fifteen days before the next menstruation. The main reason that relying on rhythm method for contraception doesn't work is that, because the number of days in the menstrual cycle isn't consistent, you can only guess at when it's fifteen days before your next period. Birth control pills prevent ovulation and override the woman's normal cycle by creating a synthetic, externally induced cycle of twenty-eight days. No ovulation, no pregnancy. The question is, how healthy is this for the normal internal cycle? Science has no answers yet. Research is sparse, and little is being done to my knowledge to investigate the issue further.

External cycles are mostly life cycles. Environmental temperature and seasonal changes, for instance, often translate into serious hormonal changes. The thyroid gland, our internal thermostat, helps us adjust to heat and cold. Modern society has altered the natural hormonal transition involved in the seasonal changes through air-conditioning and central heating. Sudden temperature shifts often affect our cycles and create problems we are not even aware of.

Becoming aware of the effect of external cycles and sudden changes becomes important in our quest to understand what throws our hormone balance off and when. The better the grasp we have of the cycle we're in at any given time, the easier it is to follow the program to keep our hormones in balance and prevent serious illness.

MEASURING HORMONES

Patients often ask, "How do I know if my hormones are balanced?"

When your hormones are in balance, you feel well. And typically, you have energy and don't crave salty or sweet foods. Your weight is stable, and your sleep pattern is consistent and uninterrupted. When you wake up in the morning, you are well rested and raring to start another day. You feel and look young and healthy.

Perhaps the above picture doesn't quite represent you. You don't feel quite that well, you suspect your hormone balance might be off, and you'd like to get a professional opinion on whether or not your hormones are in balance. Then you might ask, "How do you measure hormone balance?"

Unfortunately, present methods of testing, in my opinion, make it impossible to gain valid tests that offer realistic insights into our hormone balance. There are some blood tests that can measure individual hormones such as thyroid and testosterone. While estrogen and progesterone levels can also be measured, these measurements do not reflect the presence or absence of symptoms. We have no tests to help us extract usable information that connects blood, saliva, or urine levels of estrogen and progesterone to symptoms of hormone imbalance.

This makes it difficult, to say the least, to grasp the intricacies of balancing hormones.

Without being able to measure them or see them, how can we connect them to such obvious and unbearable problems as hot flashes, night sweats, depression, and loss of libido? The only information we can rely on comes from the medical subspecialty of endocrinology. Unfortunately, endocrinology focuses on illness, so most of the information we have is about hormonal behavior after we've become ill.

So for now, there is no scientific answer. Until reliable tests are developed and proven to work, we are left to decide on our own and with the help of our physicians whether our hormones are in balance or not. Because I have found that no existing blood, urine, or saliva test can encompass the scope of hormone fluctuations inside the human body, I believe that subjective measurement is today the only reliable method of measurement for hormone balance—in other words, it's vital to learn to read and listen to your own body's messages.

REASONABLE EXPECTATIONS

What our bodies tell us and what we want to hear are not always the same thing. We Americans are not experts at reasonable expectations. We are a nation developed from the philosophy of pushing the envelope. Many of today's health and wellness problems stem from this mentality. We believe nothing is impossible, which has allowed us to become the most highly developed country in the world, with the highest life expectancy. But we can push the limits only so far. Our bodies are not as evolved as our minds. If we want to survive into advanced age in good balance and with minimal infirmity, we must learn to listen to our bodies—within reason.

What is reasonable at fifteen may be crazy at forty. And what is reasonable to a man is not necessarily reasonable for a woman. We must learn whether our hormone balance is in concert with *reasonable expectations*. And we must understand that reasonable expectations must be considered before alterations to our hormone balance are undertaken.

᧖

Mark was sixty-eight when he came to see me. He wanted to re-gain some of the vim and vigor he had enjoyed earlier in his life. He had read about testosterone improving stamina in males and wanted to try it—not so much for sexual enhancement as to im-prove his skiing. As unusual as the request might sound, it's common for me to see patients who have specific problems that they expect hormones to solve. After evaluating his blood tests, testosterone levels, and prostate-specific antigen (PSA) levels, and receiving a clean bill of health from his primary physician, I prescribed Mark 20 mg of micronized testosterone in cream form for three months.

When he came back to see me for a two-month follow-up visit, he was ecstatic. His skiing had improved, and his sex drive had picked up speed. A blood check confirmed a rise in his testosterone levels. Mark was on a roll.

Unfortunately, his good luck came to a crashing halt halfway down a double-black-diamond slope. Mark had relied too much on hormones to improve his performance, and not enough on prac-ticing his skiing. He skied beyond his ability, broke his thighbone, and required major surgery. Recovery took six months; he lost a whole skiing season and was left with a permanent limp.

Mark is a perfect example of unreasonable expectations. Al-though testosterone was a great boost, it could not make his sixty-eight-year-old body twenty years old again. Mark should have used the improvement in his well-being to improve his muscle strength and build better resistance and balance rather than increase his speed and reckless behavior on the ski slopes.

᧖

Looking at Mark's example, we realize that balancing hormones alone is not enough. That's why the 30-Day Plan gives you more than the prescription for natural hormones you need to obtain im-provement in your hormone balance. It will help you identify and then use your personal state of homeostasis in concert with reason-able expectations to help you achieve long-lasting health, vitality, and great quality of life.

2

◌

How Your Life Affects Your Hormones and How Your Hormones Make or Break Your Life

Life changes, expected or unexpected, sudden or planned, produce shifts in hormone levels. During these shifts, symptoms develop and alter life as a whole. Understanding the connection between life changes and hormone shifts is critical to being able to adjust lifestyle, diet, exercise, and stress management to weather the storms and keep the hormones from wreaking havoc in our lives.

The key to keeping yourself in good health is often found in the anticipation of hormone changes. Knowing what to expect when changes occur may actually allow you to help prevent disease. Even small changes in the hormone balance can create a cascading effect that batters your body and mind and leads to serious illness.

Hormone changes occur all the time. For this reason alone, we would have to measure hormone levels continuously to be able to evaluate their quantitative impact on our lives. To successfully survive hormone changes, we must learn to rely on self-awareness and high levels of understanding of how our bodies function and why and how we react to change.

For starters, it is of utmost importance to fully grasp the indelible connection between hormone changes and life experiences. Change—any kind of change—creates stress. Although we are highly evolved, our stress mechanisms are old. Stress, regardless of its cause, produces the same hormonal reaction in all humans every time, a reaction that is the same as our ancestors' who lived in caves and feared attacks from bison and bear.

Stress reactions involve instant release of a series of hormones. Whether the stressor is something exciting, like going out to an amusement park, or something scary such as hearing a strange noise in the middle of the night when you are home alone, the internal reaction is always the same. Adrenaline, and then cortisol, the "flight or fight" hormones produced by the nervous system and the adrenal glands, are suddenly released. Other hormones quickly follow. The blood sugar level rises, the blood pressure is increased, your heart starts racing, and the body prepares itself to face or run from danger. Estrogen levels rise, and progesterone levels drop. The neurotransmitters fire, insulin levels spike, glucocorticoids flood the system, and blood rushes to the brain.

You are ready to fight or to run away. You get cold and clammy, you start to sweat, your palms are moist, your heartbeat is accelerating. Your thinking becomes cloudy. You start to hyperventilate.

You pass out, or you regroup and attempt to relax.

In time, if the stressor is not removed, or if you don't get used to it and stop reacting, the wear and tear on the body starts to show. Awash in cortisol, adrenaline, estrogen, insulin, and many other hormones, your system starts to wear down. You get bloated and your periods become irregular; you get acne, lose your sex drive, and become an insomniac; your moods become unpredictable; you gain weight. Your immune system gets run down, your joints begin to ache, your thinking stays foggy, you get sick, and you grow prematurely old.

Sounds awful. Yet this is what happens if we don't understand how stress—and through it hormones—affects our bodies. Once we understand what happens inside our bodies and minds at times of stress and how all these changes are intimately connected to changes in our hormones, we can take steps, such as my 30-Day Plan, to protect ourselves and limit potential long-term damage.

HORMONES AND ENVIRONMENTAL STRESSORS

Stress comes in many forms. It can come from your own body. If one organ isn't working properly, for instance, other organs become stressed out as well. But the greatest forms of stress come from outside our bodies. Much of the stress we experience every day comes directly from our environment. There are two kinds of environmental stressors that affect us: physical challenges and lifestyle changes.

THE CHALLENGES OF THE ENVIRONMENT

Since we know that everything affects our hormones, it's easy to understand that this includes everything in the environment— whether natural or human-made. Simply choosing where you live (or being born in a particular area) has a great effect on your hormones. For example, let's look at how geography affects age of onset of menstruation.

It is a well-known fact that girls who live in cold, northern climates typically start menstruating around age sixteen. Conversely, girls who live in warm climates around the equator and Tropics tend to begin to menstruate around the age of nine or ten. In temperate climates, the average age for menstruation is thirteen.

Climate and seasonal changes bring changes to our hormonal systems. If you move from one extreme climate to another, for instance, you can expect that it will take a while for your hormone system to adapt and balance itself to the new environment. Even the changes from winter to summer can cause many women to experience sudden changes in their hormone balance. In my practice, there are patients I see only when the temperature changes. Some women find hot weather intolerable, while others love it. If a change in the weather brings a dramatic change in how you feel, don't ignore it. Be even more vigilant about starting and/or sticking to the principles of the 30-Day Plan, or seek help from a health professional who is willing to comprehensively evaluate the reasons for your sudden hormonal change.

ENVIRONMENTAL HAZARDS

For all the creatures on the earth, the advances of science are both a blessing and a curse. Science has allowed us to cure or control many diseases that might have killed us all off years ago. But it has also allowed us to invent products and technologies that pollute the air and, ultimately, our bodies. Exposure to chemicals, fumes, and other environmental hazards may induce adverse hormone changes.

There are many examples of potential environmental hazards that jeopardize our hormone balance and create illnesses with dramatic and often tragic consequences. One example of serious environmental problems that are thought to be related to tragic consequences is the infamous Long Island breast cancer cluster. In 1993, the Long Island Breast Cancer Study Project was begun by the National Cancer Institute and the National Institute of Environmental Health Sciences. Although to date, statistics have failed to prove a solid connection between environmental factors and the high incidence of cancer in that area, further analysis is ongoing and scientists are still investigating the possible association between electromagnetic fields and increased risk for breast cancer. Other examples include Three Mile Island and the practice of radiating the thyroid in young children in the 1960s as a treatment for inflamed tonsils and adenoids. An article published by Dr. Arthur B. Schneider on the Internet clinical information service UpToDate in November 2002 states, "Radiation exposure of the thyroid during childhood is the most clearly defined environmental factor associated with benign and malignant thyroid tumors." While most people fortunately do not experience such radically dangerous environments, you may be particularly sensitive to even lesser hazards. Your awareness is critical to maintenance of optimum hormone balance and therefore health.

☙

Maura is forty-five and has been experiencing hot flashes, night sweats, insomnia, and loss of libido since she turned thirty-two.

She was placed on birth control pills and experienced no improvement in her symptoms. A thorough endocrine workup including magnetic resonance imaging (MRI), computerized tomography (CT) scans, X rays, blood tests, and numerous ultrasounds failed to uncover a reason for her symptoms.

When I first saw Maura, I wasn't sure there was anything more I could offer. I decided to start her on natural hormones in the hope that I could help control her symptoms in a gentler, more natural way. Searching for other ways to help, I asked Maura about her diet, exercise, and lifestyle. She ate well and exercised regularly when not completely handicapped by her symptoms. I asked about her weekend activities. Apparently, Maura felt best on Sundays and Mondays when she went biking, shopping, and spent time at home with her family.

I found the missing link when I asked Maura what type of work she did. Tuesdays through Saturdays, Maura was the hair-coloring specialist at a busy hair salon. She had started working with hair dyes at the age of thirty-two. She had never made the connection between starting her new career and the onset of her symptoms. As a test, I took her off the hormones and advised her to take a week off from work and see how she felt. Her symptoms disappeared. Within a week of her return to work, the hot flashes reappeared. I suggested to her that the chemicals she was working with might be causing her hormone imbalance. For years, obstetricians have been routinely telling their patients not to dye their hair while they are pregnant; although this is not based on scientific data, it's apparent that some people are sensitive to these types of chemicals.

Maura eventually decided to get a new job that did not involve chemical fume exposure. Although the evidence was circumstantial, she and I became convinced that the chemicals were potentially dangerous to her health. After quitting, she did not need the hormones again, and her symptoms disappeared.

≈

Maura was lucky. She discovered the specific environmental factor that was probably affecting her hormones, and was able to do something about it. Many environmental hazards, however, are unavoidable. Many people can't afford to change jobs (or move away from chemical plants or stop breathing polluted air) and must learn to make the best of difficult situations. The first step is to become aware of your surroundings. If you are not feeling well, and no medical cause has been detected, look around you. What is there in your environment that might be causing hormone imbalance? If you can, experiment by stopping the use of that substance, or by leaving the area for a short time. See if your symptoms lessen or go away completely. Once you find the probable cause, work with your doctor to find the most reasonable way to minimize the negative impact of environmental factors.

LIFESTYLE STRESSES AND HORMONAL CHANGES

When you go to most doctors' offices complaining of this, that, and the other thing, the first (and often the only) thing the doctor asks you about is your medical history. What kinds of disease have you had before? Have you ever had surgery? What medications are you taking? All these facts are important, but they leave out a whole and highly significant area of patient information. To me, such questions as "What's going on in your life right now?" and "Are you going through any changes in your life?" are just as important. After seeing patients every day for more than twenty-five years, a trend became obvious to me many years ago. Significant lifestyle environmental changes—good and bad—may be tied into changes in hormone balance.

That's because everything we do stresses us. Even starting on the 30-Day Plan, which may be a significant change for you, will cause stress. It can't be avoided. But it can be controlled, especially if you're aware that what's happening on the outside is affecting what's happening inside you.

As with physical environmental hazards, it's important to identify specific lifestyle changes that may be causing you stress. Here are some examples of outside influences that cause stress in our lives, and that we may be overlooking.

SCHOOL AND WORK

Exam Time

Not every teenager reacts the same to taking tests. But as a rule, most girls experience more PMS, acne, mood swings, and weight fluctuations. Did you ever notice how adolescent girls seem to always get their periods around exam time? Did you think it was happenstance? The reason goes back to stress and the release of cortisol during times of stress. High cortisol levels provide the signal for the pituitary gland to shut down all hormone activities that would potentially increase fertility (during times of stress, multiplying is not a high priority). The results of the messages from the pituitary gland include rapid drop in estrogen and progesterone production. This translates into getting your period. Exam time is a perfect example of why the "flight or fight" mechanism is antiquated and actually counterproductive at this time in our evolution. Exam time is not much of a threat to our lives. But it does often seem life threatening because of the hormones our body uses to react to it.

Some teens would argue that if our hormones go out of balance at exam time, it's a good reason to stop having exams, but I don't think our educational system would agree with them. We therefore need to teach our teens to protect themselves from the negative hormone changes that exam time can produce.

The first step is clearly to identify these times as potential sources of trouble to our health. The second is to implement a lifestyle, diet, and exercise program, such as the one in the 30-Day Plan, that protects us from our own biology.

Going Away to College

And you thought it was all the drinking, partying, and junk-food eating that made your teen gain weight when she went off to college? You're only partially right. Of course escape from parental control immediately translates into eating the wrong foods, drinking, and staying up all night, but if you look a little deeper into the new life your daughter is leading at college, the picture becomes more complex.

A junk-food diet, the lack of regular sleep, and the stress of being away from home add up to the same stress reaction we saw before. The human body is a beautiful mechanism, but as we already know it is limited in its ability to react to stress. From now on, stress means always the same thing—hormones out of whack.

Going away to college is a perfect example of the hormones-out-of-whack theory. The average teen comes from a caring household where meals were regular and nutritious, sleep was regular and peaceful, snacks were not permitted, exercise was encouraged and routine—and overnight this disciplined teen is set free!

With all the rules of home dismissed, what do you get?

A physical and emotional wreck who is returned to you at vacation time to put back together so she can start over again next semester.

Well, maybe I have exaggerated a little to make the point. Still, every year I see more and more college kids at vacation times when their mothers bring them to me in desperation, hoping that I can somehow return them to their precollege, early-teen health. I try to help them understand the connection between their new "free" lifestyle and their hormone-induced physical problems. I explain how improving even one of the parameters of diet, exercise, and sleep will be reflected in decreased acne, bloating, brain fog, and irregular periods.

I tell them to eat the salad bar food in the cafeteria rather than the tacos. I remind them of the waistline reduction that follows a regular workout routine and cutting back on alcohol intake. I give them vitamins and natural hormones. I ask them to start a journal. The more closely they follow the advice, the better their results. When they see how easy it is to feel better, they often take control and do it on their own.

Getting a New Job or Losing an Old One

We often spend more time at work than we do with our own families, so it's time we pay more attention to the impact work has on our well-being and on our hormones. Any significant change at work may directly affect our hormone balance. Our behavior at work, our interaction with coworkers and bosses, correlates well with our hormone balance.

When work becomes the central focus of our lives—and it often does—the balance of our hormones reflects work's impact on us. And when the conditions of work change for the better or the worse, our bodies' functions mirror them.

༃

Eleanor was twenty-six when she lost her dream job. She had spent the last four years climbing the corporate ladder. She'd always wanted to be an advertising executive. Recruited by a major New York advertising firm right out of college, she cheerfully accepted the entry-level job knowing it was the perfect start for her dream career. Within six months, she'd received a promotion, and by the time she celebrated her fourth anniversary with the company she was an assistant to one of three vice presidents. Eleanor worked hard. She rarely took time off and was always among the first to volunteer to work on weekends or holidays. She didn't have time to date or even see her family. She was committed to her career and she went to work happily every morning.

Then the economy took a turn for the worse and, like many other young people, she had no seniority. When cuts had to be made, she was among the first to go. Eleanor was crushed. By the time I saw her, almost a year later, she had been seeing a psychiatrist for her depression, had lost twenty pounds, and was borderline anorectic. She was taking two antidepressants—Celexa and Wellbutrin. Her hair was falling out, and she had moved back into her parents' house. She came to me because her periods had stopped and she was suffering with severe insomnia.

A battery of blood tests revealed a thyroid problem. Eleanor had no prior medical or other hormone problems, and as I discussed the problems with Eleanor, her internist, and her psychiatrist, the only reason we could find for the problem was the devastation the loss of the job had caused her.

I put her on the 30-Day Plan, and she did well. Her surprise at being fired and her depression at not being able to find a new job had caused her stress level to skyrocket and her hormones to go into shock. But after working with me for two months, she began to feel better. She eventually regained all the weight she had lost and went off antidepressants; her periods returned, and she learned to balance her life better. She found a new job, and two years later left to start her own public relations agency with a coworker. She got married and even started thinking about starting a family.

Retirement

Remember Lucy from the last chapter? She achieved every American's dream: She won the lottery. You'd think that life after the lottery would be sunshine and roses. It didn't turn out that way for Lucy, however, and it doesn't turn out that way for many people who face retirement. People who look forward to retirement all their lives often find the adjustment to its reality so stressful that they undergo massive hormonal shifts. Symptoms appear. Sleep becomes problematic, physical and psychological problems surface out of nowhere, accidents and illnesses suddenly impair life.

☙

Adelaide was sixty-three when she retired from her job as a travel agent. She looked forward to moving to the Carolinas and had bought a little house on the water with her daughter. The move was uneventful, so Adelaide was very surprised when she developed insomnia and night sweats within a month of her move. She had gone through menopause with no problems, and the sudden appearance of symptoms was unexpected to her. She called me, and I started her on a combination of natural hormones—estradiol and micronized progesterone—and the 30-Day Plan. Within two weeks, she felt better, and now—almost two years later—I only hear from her at Christmas, when she sends me a beautiful card.

RELATIONSHIPS

The Breakup of a Relationship

How often do young women—and older women, for that matter—experience irregular periods, skin problems, mood swings, and depression upon the breakup of a relationship? Of course you can say it's because of the trauma of the breakup. That's true, but on a physiological level, the breakup is a stressor and the woman's hormones react to the stress with the usual mechanism, which translates into significant hormone imbalance.

Research shows that many women invest their whole identity in relationships. This investment leads to severe withdrawal and stress reactions when relationships come undone.

Counseling is important to help diminish the trauma and negotiate a better self-understanding on a psychological level, but understanding how the body functions physiologically is critical to protection from long-term physical damage.

When a relationship ends, women will react strongly with hormone changes that may produce loss of appetite, depression, and changes in the regularity of periods. Estrogen and serotonin levels drop, and at times the imbalance created leads to self-medication with prescription drugs or alcohol. Understanding and acknowledging the hormonal changes associated with the breakup of a relationship and working with our body and mind in the healing process ensures complete recovery.

Getting Married

Preparing for a wedding is stressful not only because the details are endless and the pressure is on to have the perfect affair, but also because of its significant life-changing impact.

As we already know, change is perceived as stress by our bodies. Although getting married should be a happy time, the mechanisms involved are the same as in any other time of stress. In addition, many women go through major diet changes before, during, and after the wedding. What bride doesn't feel she has to lose weight for her wedding? She may go to extremes to reach what she feels is her ideal weight. After the wedding, she may gorge herself to make up for everything she has deprived herself of for months.

The honeymoon that most couples go on after the wedding is not only an opportunity for the couple to spend time alone, but should also be regarded as a recuperative period for the hormones.

Hormones and Birth Control

When Elizabeth came to see me about her hormone imbalance problems, she was twenty-seven and had been taking birth control pills for seven years. She was single and loved the security the pill gave her. She told me that she always practiced safe sex, but birth control held a very important place in her mind and she would never forgo the safety of the pill.

Unfortunately, Elizabeth had severe migraines and bloating that only got worse with the passing years. She had gone to many doctors and had changed brands of pills numerous times. Nothing helped. The headaches continued regardless.

She was reluctant to come see me because she suspected that I would immediately recommend she stop taking the pill. But her symptoms were so bad that she felt she had to give in. Elizabeth told me she expected I would place her on natural hormones. I didn't. I just took her off the birth control pills and suggested she use condoms not only as a method of practicing safe sex, but also to prevent pregnancy.

Elizabeth felt much better within a month of getting off the pill and did not need other hormonal intervention. And her headaches disappeared.

Over time, though, she did need another method of contraception because she entered a committed relationship and didn't want to continue using condoms. I recommended using an intrauterine device (IUD) without hormones in it. Many doctors are reluctant to introduce IUDs because in the 1970s, some of these devices were found to cause perforation of the uterus and/or infections that were thought to lead to infertility. Although the number of women affected was very small, the media and manufacturers of birth control pills embarked on a campaign to eliminate IUDs from the market. A study published in the *New England Journal of Medicine* in August 2001, however, refuted the link between IUDs and infertility. In fact, those researchers concluded, "Contemporary copper IUDs may be among the safest, most effective, and least expensive reversible contraceptives available." I believe that for many women current IUDs are a safe and reliable method of contraception. In Elizabeth's case, it was a little difficult to find a gynecologist to insert the IUD at first, but we ultimately managed to locate one in her native Milwaukee.

☙

Hormones in balance in our teens, twenties, and thirties make us fertile. The monthly hormone fluctuations prepare our ovaries to produce the much-cherished egg that, if fertilized by a more than willing sperm, will implant in a ready waiting uterus and produce a bouncing baby forty weeks later.

That's the role of our hormones: to perpetuate the species.

In our society, we have sex for other reasons besides having babies. Without getting too deeply involved in the politics of American sexuality, we must understand that having our hormones in balance makes us fertile, while a disruption of this delicate balance may prevent pregnancy. Birth control pills are made of synthetic substances that disrupt the balance of our own estrogen, progesterone, and testosterone and prevent ovulation. These pills are harsh intruders into a young woman's body chemistry and her natural hormone balance. Although they do effectively accomplish the task of disrupting normal hormone balance, thus preventing ovulation, they also disrupt other functions and often create undesirable side effects, such as bloating, mood swings, depression, loss of libido, weight gain, and acne.

Numerous papers and scientific research studies, sponsored

primarily by the manufacturers of birth control pills, claim that
birth control pills may be used safely. These papers refute connections between prolonged usage of birth control pills and infertility,
cancer, depression, mood swings, or migraines.

In my twenty-five years of clinical practice involved with caring
for young women, I have encountered all too many who experience
serious and long-lasting side effects while on birth control pills
(mentioned above) that have made me question the validity and
reliability of these studies. I therefore use the following guidelines,
based on my experience with my patients over twenty-five years,
when I give advice on methods of birth control:

- If the patient has no side effects from taking birth control pills
  after three months, it's generally fine to stay on them for a maximum of one year at a time, then take a break for a few months.
  I don't prescribe them for more than three years. There are many
  studies under way that continue to explore the effects of long-
  term use of birth-control pills, but definitive conclusions haven't
  yet been reached. I advise my patients to be on the safe side, and
  use them for shorter periods of time.
- I prescribe the lowest-content synthetic hormones birth control
  pills possible.
- I'm loath to use the newest birth control pill on the market as
  soon as it comes out; wait for it to develop a track record of reliability and safety before jumping on its bandwagon.

I also suggest using nonhormonal methods of birth control:

- **IUDs** (without hormones) are relatively safe and underutilized
because of bad publicity more than twenty years ago. There has
been reluctance to insert IUDs in women who have never had a
child. Their side effects—typically heavy periods and cramps—are
tolerable for most users.

- **Diaphragms** are not as reliable a method of contraception as
the IUD. If care is taken to fill the diaphram with contraceptive gel
every time you have sex, it is as effective as birth control pills and
it doesn't have systemic effects. Many of my patients complain that
it is messy, awkward to insert, and occasionally difficult to remove.

The only known side effects are occasional allergies to the contraceptive gel. Recurring vaginal infections are also sometimes encountered.

- **Cervical caps.** Rarely used, they cover the cervical opening and prevent sperm from entering into the uterus. Problems revolve around them being cumbersome and difficult to insert and remove.
- **Condoms.**
- **Foams.** Chemical spermicidal foams inserted in the vagina before intercourse are unreliable, and the failure rate is very high. They provide no protection from sexually transmitted diseases.
- **Rhythm method.** Using a basal temperature thermometer, you take your temperature every day and then avoid sex for forty-six to seventy-two hours after the temperature spike that represents ovulation. It is a quite safe and reliable method—if you take your basal temperature faithfully the second you wake up every morning. Most people, however, are not as faithful as they should be, and unwanted pregnancy is often the result. These days, the rhythm method is used more often to get pregnant than to avoid it.

Having a Baby

The hormonal changes involved in the process of having a baby were covered in detail in *The Hormone Solution*. The whole pregnancy process is about ever-increasing and changing hormones, the interaction of which provides the necessary environment for the development and growth of the fetus.

During the forty weeks of pregnancy, hormone levels are astronomical and constantly on the rise. The woman's body undergoes incredible changes. Nine months is a long time, and our bodies become awash in hormones whose effects vary from making us feel highly sexual, immortal, beautiful, and positively glowing to feeling fat and ugly, bloated, fatigued, totally disinterested in sex, and miserable. Our ability to think is impaired one day, while the next we are mental giants.

Hormonal changes leave us exhausted and unable to move from bed to chair the first trimester, than cause us to be brimming with energy the last few weeks before birth, nesting, cleaning, and preparing the home for the new arrival. It's important for both the mother and the father to realize that these fluctuations are the normal results of hormonal changes. Following a healthy lifestyle at this time of life is more important than ever to keep the hormone changes within reasonable limits without harming the growth and development of the baby or negatively affecting the mother's well-being.

After Childbirth

We are familiar with postpartum blues, postpartum depression, and the rare but devastating postpartum psychosis. All these clinical diagnoses are directly connected to issues of hormone balance. The stress of the delivery followed by the stress of having a newborn, new family structure, loss of freedom, and changes in body image and shape are reflected in the balance of hormones that completely changes after childbirth.

Unfortunately, too many doctors ignore women's postpartum complaints or are uneducated about the significant role of hormone disruption after childbirth. They are likely to tell new mothers to simply wait it out, that the postpartum blues will disappear on their own. More often than not, the hormones do get back to a balanced state by themselves. But if the depression continues or worsens after several weeks, be sure to let your doctor know—or find one who will focus on helping you get your hormones back on track.

Divorce

Another life change that produces an enormous amount of stress is divorce. It isn't uncommon for me to see women in their midforties to fifties going into traumatic menopause during divorce proceedings.

Lucinda is a fifty-three-year-old schoolteacher with two grown children away in college. I've known her for more than ten years. She had no major medical problems and came to see me for annual physicals and flu shots. I didn't know much about her personal life, except that she was married to a successful businessman. One early spring, Lucinda arrived for her appointment disheveled and drawn.

She couldn't sleep or eat; she had night sweats and hot flashes. She was unable to focus at work, and at home she had no interest in keeping house. She had no idea why. Ready to start a thorough workup, I asked about any changes in her home or work situations. Casually she said her husband had left home. Her demeanor was disconnected—she spoke as if she were talking about a third party. Prompted by my questions, Lucinda told me her marriage had never been a "match made in heaven." She and her husband had "an arrangement and divorce was not an option. And then one day, he changed the rules. He left."

The shock of the change, while a surprise to Lucinda, was an even bigger surprise to her hormones. She went into what is medically referred to as traumatic menopause. Her master gland, the pituitary, ordered the whole system to shut down, and she suddenly went into ovarian failure and thus hormone depletion.

⌘

This is not an unusual situation. Many women, no matter what their age, enter menopause due to traumatic experiences. Thus, if you're going through a divorce or experiencing any type of stressful, traumatic situation, this is the time to look at your hormone balance and use the 30-Day Plan to help you weather the storm.

Death of a Loved One

The emotional stress of losing a loved one is covered in every psychiatry textbook. Unfortunately, the connection between emotional loss and hormone changes has received very little study.

⌘

Monique was thirty-four when her mother, Katherine, suddenly died. Katherine had been a big help to Monique, emotionally and physically. She baby-sat for Monique's three-month-old daughter, which allowed Monique to return to work as a bank teller.

Monique became emotionally paralyzed by her mother's untimely death. She could not get out of bed and could not stop crying. She lost interest in the baby and in life in general. She stopped having periods and stopped eating.

She saw a psychiatrist, who placed her on Wellbutrin and Concerta. She took Valium to sleep at night. She drank coffee and smoked cigarettes constantly throughout the day. The more medication she was placed on, the worse she got. Her face became covered with acne, and her weight loss was of serious concern.

When I saw Monique, her psychiatrist had just recommended hospitalization. She didn't want to leave her baby and came to me ready to do anything. I started her on natural progesterone, the supplement program, and eliminated all coffee and cigarettes from her diet. I asked her to follow the detoxification part of the 30-Day Plan for two weeks. I also asked her to take a twenty-minute walk every day. She followed the program and stayed on it for the following six months. She did not require hospitalization. She stopped taking Concerta by the second month of the program and Wellbutrin by the fourth. Her symptoms disappeared over a month's time.

Two years later, she still cried every time she spoke of her mother. But she was able to go on with her life. Her child is happy and healthy, Monique herself has returned to her normal weight, and she finds enormous joy in taking care of the baby herself. She has chosen not to return to work, and her husband has been very supportive. They still go to therapy together, and she tells me her marriage is stronger than ever.

༄

Monique was depressed by her mother's sudden death and overwhelmed by the responsibility of a newborn baby. Her physical symptoms resonated with the status of her hormones. In my opinion, hospitalizing her would have been a potentially dangerous move. Removing her from her baby and husband would have only created more imbalance in her life.

She needed integration into her life while experiencing the loss and allowing time and medical and psychiatric intervention to help her heal.

MEDICAL STRESSES

Surgery and Illness

Not every illness is caused by hormone imbalance, but every illness causes significant hormone balance changes. Illness is a reaction to lowered immune function. Hormone fluctuations directly affect immune function and recovery. During times of illness, sleep, diet, and exercise regimens become even more important than usual because they directly affect recovery.

Surgery has often been associated with changes in menstrual cycle regularity and even sudden menopause. A small study of ten young women undergoing breast operations in Europe revealed that the time of surgery precipitated onset of their periods.

When I was a resident at Kings County Hospital, in New York, we brought pads to the recovery room routinely for young women who underwent surgical procedures. Many women got their periods after a surgical procedure even if the period was not due.

My mother was forty-six when she had a kidney removed because of a persistent infection that could not be cured with antibiotics. When she went into surgery, she had her period. When she came out, her period had stopped and never returned. She went into traumatic menopause. It was never addressed by any physician. I know the story because I asked my mother about her menstrual history in order to learn more about my own genetic predisposition. I found the story fascinating because traumatic menopause is often encountered in our time among women experiencing severe illnesses, operations, or emotional trauma. These women may or may not experience other symptoms of menopause after the sudden disappearance of their periods. My mother did not, and the story of her last period only surfaced when I became an expert in hormones and started asking questions.

To this day I wonder why our mothers' generation had so little trouble with menopause while our generation and those following are becoming so handicapped by ever-increasing numbers of symptoms. Were the symptoms there and ignored, or are these symptoms another evolutionary change?

Run-Down Immune System

The state of our immune system reflects fluctuations in hormone levels. Immune deficiency syndromes such as HIV/AIDS, cancers, and severe infections are invariably associated with symptoms of hormone imbalance. How often do you find that around your period, you are more vulnerable to colds, headaches and migraines, intestinal problems, or allergies? You probably don't pay much attention to these connections, yet if you do, you can do something to avoid these things. You can get more sleep, improve your diet, run around less, and take a few extra vitamins and supplements (which I will detail in chapter 7) around that time of the month. This is the perfect time to go on the 30-Day Plan to balance your hormones and protect yourself from a run-down immune system.

Menopause

Because menopause is such a hot topic, it would be easy to assume everyone knows and understands the connection between menopause and hormone imbalances.

When I started working with hormones, my practice was limited to menopausal women. Instead of spending my time addressing issues of hormone imbalance, educating and offering solutions, I found myself defending my peers. The women I saw were angry and bitterly disappointed with the conventional medical system.

They felt that the physicians who'd delivered their babies and had supposedly known them for decades were suddenly unable to help and, even worse, were unwilling to listen. They offered no solutions or help to women who were undergoing traumatic physical and mental transformations no one had prepared them for. Somehow menopause was a plague, a time in life when either the woman or the problems were discarded or blatantly ignored. Adding insult to injury, most physicians offered no treatment until a woman had had no menstrual period for one year, regardless of how severe the symptoms were before that arbitrarily chosen point in time.

In 1983, I was the director of the emergency department at Westchester County Medical Center in suburban New York. I was in my early thirties and I knew little about menopause. Medical textbooks and therapeutic manuals did not address it.

One day, I saw a woman in the ER. Her husband brought her in. He said, "She snapped." She had been seeing a psychiatrist who had placed her on a then-popular antidepressant, but according to the husband she was still crazy. When I asked what the problem was, he told me, "She doesn't listen to me anymore and she doesn't want to cook and clean or take care of the kids. She wants to go back to school and become a nurse." Didn't sound crazy to me.

Maybe twenty years ago, a woman entering menopause and looking for fulfillment outside the house was unusual. Today it's the norm. And tomorrow we may actually support and encourage women to change and expand their lives before they reach menopause.

I sent them both home. Unfortunately, I had no solutions for either one of them. I told the husband the wife was not crazy, she was just trying to find herself. He probably thought I was crazy, and I wasn't even menopausal. He left in a huff and swore he would never go to a woman doctor again.

Today I have many reliable and excellent solutions (which you'll discover as you read the rest of the book). The 30-Day Plan offers a combination of the safest and most successful cutting-edge solutions available for problems of menopause and hormone imbalances available today. This plan looks at you as a whole person, an individual with needs and fears not to be discarded or ignored. All you have to do is take the opportunity offered and implement it in your life.

THE MIND–BODY CONNECTION

Hormones and Mental Health

When I was going to medical school, I loved every psychiatry course I took. I have always been interested in mental health, and even though I did not feel compelled to become a psychiatrist, I firmly believed no physician could be successful at her practice if she didn't understand the psychology of her patients.

Over the last three decades, research has emerged firmly establishing the involvement of hormones in practically every chemical reaction in the body. As the data accumulate and become further validated by experiments, the balance of hormones appears to directly affect physical and mental presentation of increasing numbers of problems in medicine.

In the 1980s, a surgeon by the name of Bernie Siegel left his booming surgical practice to work with cancer patients through nonsurgical methods. This decision was looked down upon by many medical professionals. Dr. Siegel's research prompted him to state unequivocally that there was a direct connection between cancer outcome and the psychology of the patient. He dedicated his life to teaching patients to reach into their minds to accomplish cures that surgeons could not. His popular book *Love, Medicine & Miracles* prompted many in the medical establishment to write a slew of retaliatory articles in the medical journals trying to dispel any possible connection between illnesses (cancer in this case), their treatments or cures, and the mind.

I read Bernie Siegel's books with great interest and excitement. I had been a trauma doctor and an internist for almost ten years by the time they were published. I always thought there was much more to a medical or surgical outcome than the medication or the procedure. I saw some patients die for no reason and saw others survive against all odds.

I had no clinical studies or scientific literature to back up my observations. I had an empirical, gut feeling that there was a significant connection between mind and body, but medicine does not encourage gut feelings.

Ten years later, in 1989, I took a look at the progress of fifty patients in my internal medicine practice over a period of three years. The general statistics at the time for a practice comparable to mine in age, gender, and socioeconomic level revealed that a norm of one in ten (meaning five in the group I looked at) would experience some kind of severe illness and or hospitalization over this period. My patients had undergone no hospitalizations or major surgeries. There are innumerable variables in everything we do. Scientific data are always skewed and never reflect an unbiased situation. In my small retrospective review, the difference between what was expected and what occurred was most likely due to my approach to treating the patient as a whole, not as a disease. Of course I treated the headache, flu, high blood pressure, or irritable bowel, but that was never the only thing I treated. Integrating all aspects of the patient's life worked wonders to improve outcome and get the patients on their feet faster. Initially, I thought it was just blind luck that made me get healthier patients. Eventually, I learned that it wasn't. Treating the whole person is, I now believe, the only way to practice medicine to achieve success.

Unequivocally and indelibly connected, our hormones and mental health can no longer be separated. Serotonin, whose levels in the brain determine how happy or miserable we are, is a hormone. Serotonin levels parallel estrogen levels and are modulated by progesterone. Cortisol and insulin, two other extremely important hormones, also directly affect serotonin levels.

During my medical training years, at Kings County Hospital and at Downstate in Brooklyn, New York, I learned nothing about integrating medical problems, hormone imbalances, and psychological issues. There were two psychiatrists, however—Drs. Norman Levy and Michael Blumenfield—who ran a department called liaison psychiatry. It was their mission to make connections between a particular patient's illness and his or her mental state, relationships, and environmental problems. The two psychiatrists made rounds on the medical floors with a group of medical students in tow, asking the patients about their family life, their relationships, and their family histories. They then made the most remarkable connections between the patients' personality, lifestyle, and background, and the illness that had brought them to the hospital.

I was fascinated by their work. I learned more about taking a complete history and looking at a person as a whole from them than from anyone else in my entire medical training. Mental health is the result of a combination of genetics, hormone balances and interactions, and life. So when considering depression, mood swings, or seasonal affective disorders, we mustn't limit our search to mental issues and overlook the connection to our whole system and our hormones.

Dr. Michael Blumenfield, the psychiatrist I spoke of earlier, has written a book called *Consultation-Liaison Psychiatry* (Lippincott Williams & Wilkins, 2003; cowritten with Maria L. A. Tiamson, part of the Practical Guides in Psychiatry series). Every page of this manual, directed at teaching psychiatrists to integrate medical problems with psychiatric issues, is a testimonial to the connections between mind and body. The specialty of liaison psychiatry is alive and well, and pioneers such as Dr. Blumenfield continue their quest to make physicians and the public aware humans, functioning as whole beings.

Hormones and Sleep

You may think that all we get when we sleep is rest. This could not be farther from the truth. While we sleep, our body is busy manufacturing hormones. It is only during those few quiet seven or eight hours during the night that the human organism does something it cannot do any other time—build hormones.

If these hours of rest do not occur, our bodies don't make enough hormones to keep us from getting sick, getting foggy, becoming depressed and moody, or growing hypoglycemic and snappy. So when you decide to skip another night of sleep to party, or work, or go to the gym to keep those muscles buff instead of getting eight hours of shuteye, remember, you are depleting your hormones and damaging your body and mind.

That's why I personally will not give up the struggle to teach teenagers that sleep is the only thing that will make up for the lost nights of partying at college. I will also never acquiesce to the thirty-year-olds who invariably try to convince me that if they don't finish a project on time their whole career will end, which makes them forgo sleep but not partying.

The need for sleep is critical in the hormone renewal and manufacturing process. As we age, regardless of how well we diet, exercise, supplement, or deal with stress, the quality of our sleep diminishes. Sleep disturbances are most prevalent in the aging population, the group with the diminishing hormone levels.

If our hormones are out of balance, we find ourselves not sleeping well, not getting rested, feeling worn down and fatigued at all times. This situation is a dirty trick Mother Nature plays on us. When we are no longer needed to produce children or raise them, we stop being able to sleep. We have to trick Mother Nature into believing we are young again by replenishing some of those hormone levels with the help of diet, exercise, natural hormones, and supplements.

September 11, 2001

This devastating event in our country's history had far-reaching effects, including many on the general population's mind–body connection. For six months following September 11, 2001, I volunteered at a local New York TV station answering call-ins from shell-shocked New Yorkers. The pain and devastation were palpable, and the work of healing I believed I was engaging in proved more than I knew how to handle.

I couldn't sleep for months, I had hot flashes and night sweats, and I walked around in a brain fog. My hormones were responding to a never-before-experienced trauma. During those six months, I listened to and saw women from all walks of life with similar symptoms. Most of them had experienced no direct loss and felt guilty about feeling sick and taking up my time. Slowly we all learned to accept and understand the changes our bodies were undergoing, and I was able to help women connect their symptoms of hormone imbalances to the trauma we had all experienced. Even if direct loss had not occurred, the communal loss affected every one of us, and our bodies reacted the only way they knew: through our hormone balance.

A year after September 11, I returned to the New York TV station for a two-week call-in show in preparation for the anniversary of the tragic day. I worked with psychiatrists and psychologists who were experts on emotional reactions to stress. No one was prepared for the physical fallout of the tragedy. One year later, women with insomnia, night sweats, mood disorders, hot flashes, menstrual problems, and loss of libido were still reacting hormonally. This time we were able to make the connection with hormones more easily and offer a more comprehensive type of treatment.

BONE DEFICIENCIES, HEART DISEASE, AND OTHER PHYSICAL RESULTS OF HORMONE IMBALANCE

With all the stress factors above, plus many more I have not listed, it's a wonder any of us makes it to old age. When we do make it to our seventies and eighties, many of us are plagued with chronic illnesses. We dread the aging process not only because we live in a youth-oriented culture and don't want to lose the appearance of youth, but also because we fear chronic illnesses and infirmity. The thought of being at the mercy of a caretaker is enough of a motivator for most of us to do whatever it takes to avoid dependency at all cost.

Our whole medical establishment and the pharmaceutical industry were developed around this enormous fear of chronic illness and disability. While advancements in medicine have helped extend our lives and brought us drugs and surgical modalities to keep us functional into our twilight years, the system has failed to deliver the true preventive solutions.

It is in the realm of alternative and integrative medicine that we find the lifestyle issues seriously and successfully addressed. Conventional medicine can and will treat your acute problems, but it will not provide you with a system for quick recovery after surgery or help you reintegrate into an active and productive life after a serious illness.

Conventional medicine generally focuses on finding disease and then developing medication to treat it. Sometimes this approach overlooks the importance of preventing disease and staying healthy.

OSTEOPOROSIS

Take osteoporosis, for instance. Bones are constantly being made and destroyed in our bodies under the direction of multiple hormones. Hormones are responsible for the mechanisms by which calcium and other minerals are pushed into the cells that make bones. Hormone balance determines the rate of construction versus destruction they continuously undergo. With the aging process and the subsequent depletion of hormones in our bodies, the process of making bones decreases and the process of destroying bones dominates the picture.

Before alendronate sodium (marketed as Fosamax) and risedronate (marketed as Actonel), medications that help stop bone destruction (but do not improve bone thickness), osteoporosis was generally a diagnosis made at autopsy on old people or people with seriously defective hormone balances. Only after these drugs arrived on the market did osteoporosis rise to public consciousness.

Progress is wonderful, but scaring women and now even men about the dangers of a new so-called disease of aging just because we found a drug to potentially treat it with poses an ethical problem for me. Before the advent of Fosamax, no statistical data on the significance of osteoporosis in younger people existed. Until Merck (the company that makes Fosamax) started investigating the effects of Fosamax on bone mass, there were virtually no studies on the incidence and frequency of osteoporosis or fractures in younger women.

I believe in the importance of medical evolution. And I believe we need information on the significance of thinning bones. We need prospective studies that determine the real connection between thin bones and incidence of fractures. We need to be able to correlate the significance of osteopenia and osteoporosis to numbers of fractures caused by these conditions. Until these studies are performed, however, I believe that we are in the dark. Osteopenia may or may not progress to osteoporosis, and osteoporosis may or may not cause increased incidence of fractures in younger women. Taking Fosamax can increase the density and thickness of your bones, but the long-term side effects of the drug are still unknown. It has been on the market for less than ten years. It has been associated with problems of the kidneys and liver, and blood tests must be taken on patients at regular intervals to ensure that the drug is not producing adverse reactions.

Calcium supplementation is a more benign option, but it, too, can be fraught with problems. There are hundreds of calcium preparations on the market. They are not all the same. The type of calcium you decide to take makes a difference. Most preparations do not enter our bones, so the calcium we take goes right through the body and is excreted in the urine or becomes a kidney stone.

Calcium orotate and arginate, in which calcium is attached to an amino acid, are two types of calcium supplements scientifically proven to absorb well into the cells. The problem with these preparations is that they are very expensive—and often, even if the label does say the calcium is attached to the amino acid, it doesn't get absorbed in the combination. Do not despair, though.

Use a good combination of calcium and magnesium (magnesium and zinc in addition to vitamin D supplementation improve calcium absorption) if you are having difficulty finding or affording the amino acid calcium supplements, and take it at night when the hormones that increase bone production become active. I believe that following my plan is more likely to help prevent osteoporosis without side effects than any drug. In my opinion, the primary situation under which you should consider taking Fosamax today is if you have a family history of osteoporosis and family members who had fractures at early ages. Otherwise, you may want to follow the 30-Day Plan and:

- Eat right.
- Increase your activity level.
- Avoid running or exercises that pound down on your joints and bones as you age.
- Perform strength-building exercises daily.
- Address imbalances of your hormones with natural hormones.
- Check your thyroid and parathyroid hormone levels and make sure they are well balanced.
- Take supplements that protect your bones and improve your body's ability to synthesize hormones.

HEART DISEASE

For decades, heart disease was considered exclusively a disease of men in their middle years. Then in the 1990s, the Heart and Estrogen/Progestin Replacement Study I (HERS I) uncovered the fact that women after menopause have the same incidence of heart disease as men. Sad but true, the statistical incidence of heart disease in postmenopausal women rises sharply to equal the incidence of heart disease in men. The sudden rise in heart disease has been connected to the loss of hormones women experience at menopause. Estrogen, found in abundance in young women, provides them significant protection against heart disease. The loss of estrogen with aging and with recurrent episodes of hormone imbalance can help eliminate this protection, contributing to increases in serum cholesterol levels, in atherosclerotic plaques deposited into the lining of the arteries—and in the risk of heart disease.

If you look at statistics, it appears as though the risk of heart disease suddenly quadruples in menopausal women. This is misleading. The incidence of heart disease is indeed higher in postmenopausal women. But estrogen doesn't just leave our system one day, and *poof*—we get heart disease the next. It's a slow and steady process.

We have decades to prepare for the day our hormones leave, and we have a lifetime to develop protective lifestyles, eating habits, and exercise programs. Instead of becoming scared at the prospect of getting heart disease and being intimidated by statistical data and overzealous reporting on the topic, let's start protecting ourselves from this risk now. By following the 30-Day Plan from the time we are in our twenties, we will prevent heart disease long before it starts.

Hormone imbalance and depletion accelerates the appearance and progression of chronic illness. There is no doubt that besides hormones, other important factors contribute to aging and infirmity, but if we are successful at keeping our hormones in balance we diminish the negative effects of other influences.

WHERE DO GENETICS FIT INTO THE PICTURE?

The bulk of this chapter has focused on outside influences and how they affect our bodies and our hormones. The degree of that effect, and the form it takes, is often determined by the way we are genetically programmed.

We are what our genetic material has provided us with. We must learn to understand our genetics, accept them, and use them to our benefit. We can then use this knowledge to protect us from what is ahead.

When your doctor asks you about your family history, he/she's looking at your genetics. What happened to your parents, grandparents, and practically all blood relatives presents a preview of what diseases you are likely to develop as you age, and what your risk factors are.

ᔐ

When Mauro came to see me, he was forty-five and worried. His father had died of a massive coronary at the same age, and Mauro did not relish the same fate. Unfortunately, Mauro had not paid attention to his genetics. He was overweight, a heavy smoker and drinker, a junk-food eater, and a couch potato to boot. The odds were against him. I would have loved to say to him: *Mauro, if you had watched your diet, exercised, and stopped smoking and drinking twenty years ago, you would have probably beaten the odds. You might have outsmarted your genetics.* Instead, I told him that it was never too late to start taking control of his life. The last thing I wanted was to add more stress to a dangerous situation. So I started with the smoking and the diet. He had a thorough medical workup that included a cardiac stress test, which he thankfully passed. I gave Mauro testosterone and progesterone, supplements, and vitamins to protect and enhance his hormone balance.

I followed him carefully for six months. He started exercising, improved his diet, and lost forty pounds. He became an avid tennis player and stopped being a couch potato. He is now fifty-four, and the best part about his story is that he teaches his coworkers how to help prevent illness by paying attention to family history in their twenties and thirties and starting preventive measures early.

౼ఌ

Do not wait. All you have is today. Armed with knowledge about your genetic predispositions, you can help start preventing disease today!

3

◯

The Natural Hormone Solution:
What Are the Alternatives to Synthetics?

When I wrote *The Hormone Solution*, I toyed with naming it *The* Natural *Hormone Solution*. The reason I didn't was because of the medical perception of the word *natural* at that time. Although the public has always been positive toward everything natural, the medical profession shied away from the term.

While the public believes *natural* translates into "protective, pure and clean, helping to prevent illness and maintain well-being," the medical profession considers it to mean "unproven witchcraft." *Natural* was reserved for alternative medical practices and therapies, herbal remedies, and old wives' tales. Unfortunately, this mind-set eliminated natural hormones from the conventional medical consciousness—and from the title of my book.

This book is a different story, however. Many factors, including the results of the National Institutes of Health study revealing harmful effects of synthetic hormone replacements, have opened the door to acceptability for natural hormones to physicians and consumers alike. And unlike many products in the alternative market, natural hormone products are regulated by the Food and Drug Administration.

Here are the names you'll become most familiar with when learning about natural hormones:

Natural Estrogens

- Estradiol.
- Estriol.
- Estrone.

Natural Progesterone

- Micronized progesterone.

Natural Testosterone

- Micronized testosterone.

WHY SHOULD YOU USE NATURAL HORMONES?

Natural hormones are an FDA-approved class of products, mass-produced by pharmaceutical companies and on the market for more than twenty years. They're called "natural" hormones and classified as "bioidentical" because biologically they are identical to human hormones. Their chemical formulas are identical in structure to the steroid sex hormones produced by our bodies. This is not the case with synthetic hormones.

Natural hormones are made from plants (such as yams and soy) and mimic the chemical structure of the human hormone. Natural hormones are the closest in chemical structure, actions, and inter-action to those hormones produced by humans.

Whether estrogens or progesterone, natural hormones do not interfere with, displace, or replace human hormones. Therefore, their action is gentle, and they are read by the human body (cell receptors) as part of its own. Because they are the only types of hormones that look exactly like the hormones our body makes, they are less likely to cause adverse reactions. When you have substances like natural hormones that are readily available, why would you even consider synthetics?

In my experience with patients on the 30-Day Plan, I found that women taking synthetic hormone replacement therapy (HRT) or birth control pills in conjunction with the program did not obtain the same benefits as those women using natural hormones. Synthetic HRT and birth control pills have numerous side effects, cited in previous chapters (bloating, swollen breasts, weight gain, mood swings, and loss of libido), which can drain your system instead of improving your hormone balance. If you use birth control pills or other synthetic hormones while on the program, your body may be spending much of its time fighting their negative side effects. All the components of the 30-Day Plan are designed to work in concert to promote an ideal hormone balance. It is counterproductive to include medications that detract from the overall goal.

THE MOLECULAR FORMULA OF NATURAL/BIOIDENTICAL HORMONES

It's important to look briefly at the molecular structure of progesterone and estradiol, the two main sex hormones we work with when balancing our hormones in the 30-Day Plan.

PROGESTERONE

In the diagram on page 53, the formula for human progesterone is on the right; on the left is natural progesterone. They are exactly the same. In the middle I have placed the formula of the synthetic progestin used in Prempro and Provera. Notice the three CH_3 groups (in boldface). They clearly create a different molecule from the ones of natural and human progesterone.

Once introduced into the human body, the synthetic hormone might fool the body into believing that it's progesterone—very unlikely due to its formula—or it might create adverse reactions. When we have the option of natural progesterone with an identical chemi-

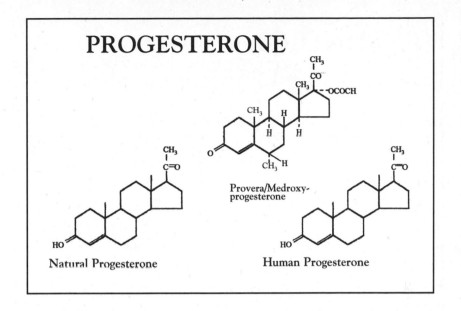

PROGESTERONE

Provera/Medroxy-progesterone

Natural Progesterone

Human Progesterone

cal formula to our own, why would we ever consider putting foreign synthetic substances into our bodies? I have asked this question of more than five hundred patients in the past year. The only answer I received was, "I didn't know." Once people are informed and understand the difference between synthetics and naturals, they tend to choose the natural route.

ESTRADIOL

I am often asked why I use estradiol rather than estriol or estrone, the other component molecules of estrogen. Here's why: Estriol is most abundant in pregnancy and is considered a weak estrogen, with little evidence supporting its beneficial use in aging women. Estriol is found in high concentrations in the placenta and has been found to provide mucosal lining improvement in the vaginas of older women. In the mid-1990s, a few reports emerged on its use as a selective cardio protector. The data were not duplicated.

Estrone is dominant in perimenopausal years, has been linked to breast cancer, and is already present in aging woman. I believe supplementing it increases the risks that endogenous estrogen poses as we age.

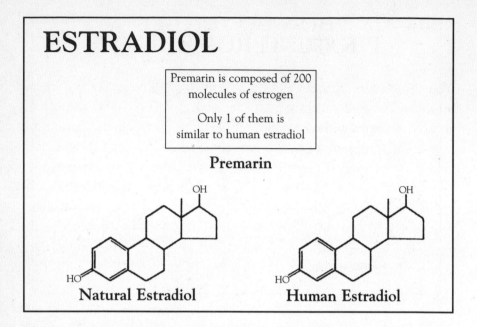

ESTRADIOL

Premarin is composed of 200 molecules of estrogen

Only 1 of them is similar to human estradiol

Premarin

OH

HO

Natural Estradiol

OH

HO

Human Estradiol

Estradiol, the one I favor, is the most abundant estrogen in young women in their twenties who are at their peak health—sexually, physically, and mentally.

Our goal in the implementation of the 30-Day Plan is to maintain youthful hormone balance. That's why I rely on estradiol, the estrogen of youth, to help keep us young.

Look at the molecular formula of estradiol above. On the right is the formula of human estradiol; on the left, natural estradiol. They look exactly the same. Thus, no adverse reaction should be expected in the human body. Let's now turn to the box in the middle. It describes the chemical formula of the most often prescribed synthetic estrogen replacement medication, Premarin.

Premarin, also known as conjugated equine estrogens, is made of two hundred various molecules derived from pregnant horse's urine. Only one of these two hundred molecules resembles the molecular structure of estradiol.

HOW DO YOU GET
NATURAL HORMONES?

You can obtain natural progesterone at the health food store in low strengths (called subtherapeutic in medical lingo) and sometimes in combination with other herbal products, supplements, and vitamins. The problem with the over-the-counter preparations is their inability to reach therapeutic levels in our system. In other words, they don't provide enough active hormones to help us feel significantly better over the long term. Natural hormones in over-the-counter preparations not only contain low concentrations of progesterone but also contain no estrogens, because estrogen cannot be dispensed without prescription.

PHYTOESTROGENS

Some herbs have estrogen-like effects. Called phytoestrogens, they're surrounded by controversy and little sound scientific data.

Phytoestrogens are plant-derived combinations of products that have estrogen-like effects. Proponents of phytoestrogens maintain that they are efficacious and safe, while their adversaries suggest an association with increased cancer risk. The issue at the core of the debate is that phytoestrogens mimic some of the actions of estrogen on the body, but because they are not true estrogens, they mask potentially significant warning signs of estrogen imbalance. Scientific data on phytoestrogens are sparse even though it is a thriving multimillion-dollar industry.

They have become very popular since you don't need a prescription for them, and because they provide a certain comfort level to women who are scared of synthetic hormones and cannot seem to find physicians knowledgeable and willing to work with natural hormones. But since they may mask symptoms of hormone imbalance, they may be giving a false sense of security to those who use them.

Until reliable scientific research is conducted and more information becomes available on phytoestrogens, I don't advise my patients to take them for prolonged periods. If you do use them, I advise diligent medical supervision and follow-up with regular mammograms and pelvic ultrasounds. The products available under the category of phytoestrogens include but are not limited to:

- Estroven.
- Bio-PMT.
- Energenics.
- Flavonoids and bioflavonoids.

They all contain combinations of herbs, many of which would benefit from more clinical data substantiating the claims of safety and efficacy behind them.

HORMONE PRECURSORS

Another category of over-the-counter products with potential impact on your hormone balance is called hormone precursors. Precursors are substances that exist in the human body naturally and may transform into hormones under specific circumstances. The key to their efficacy is their actual transformation.

Hypothetically, these substances could provide necessary substrates, the skeleton upon which the human body could manufacture hormones. But to accomplish this transformation, specific sequences of events must occur. The precursor must be absorbed into the system, then it must become available for interaction with other substances, and then appropriate chemical reactions must occur to facilitate the manufacture of proper hormones. The problem with taking over-the-counter hormone precursor preparations is that there are no guarantees for their absorption into our bodies, their bioavailability to our cells, or their transformation into active hormones.

Examples of these hormone precursors are:

- Dihydro-epiandrosterone (DHEA).
- Pregnenelone.
- MediTropin.
- PROhGH.
- Secretagogues.
- Somatotropin.

All hormone precursors are available over the counter. Since there are no reliable tests to measure their bioavailability in the body, we are left to decide their usefulness on an individual case-by-case basis. As with the phytoestrogens, my advice is to try them only under the supervision of your doctor, who may recommend that you stay on them only for a short period of time. See how you feel before you embark on a long and expensive relationship with hormone precursors. See how you feel after one month. If your symptoms improve, your doctor may recommend that you continue; and if he/she doesn't, either change to a combination of supplements and vitamins (see chapter 7) that help your own body make the much-needed hormones or have your doctor prescribe natural hormones.

Warning: If you are using phytoestrogens or hormone precursors, do not use them together with any prescription natural hormones or others, with synthetics, or with birth control pills.

NATURAL HORMONE PREPARATIONS

The following preparations are available at drugstores and pharmacies by prescription from your physician.

Natural Estrogen Patches

- Alora.
- Climara.
- FemPatch.
- Menorest.

- Vivelle-Dot/Vivelle.
- Estraderm.
- Esclim.
- Estrace.

Natural Estrogen Tablets

- Estradiol.
- Biestrogen (Biest).
- Estrace.
- Triestrogen (Triest).
- Estriol.

Natural Progesterone

- Prometrium.
- Progesterone gel.
- Progesterone cream.
- Oral micronized progesterone.

Looking at these lists, you'll notice that estrogen and progesterone preparations available through a commercial source, by prescription only, at your local pharmacy are separated. There is no commercially available natural hormone product on the market as of this writing that combines natural estrogen with natural progesterone. In my opinion, this is a serious oversight that leaves a gaping hole in the use of natural hormones to balance public needs.

From our Hormones 101 course, we know that estrogen and progesterone work together. It isn't the individual hormone level that makes us feel good or bad, it's the combination—the interaction among hormones—that helps us reach and maintain homeostasis. Combining the two hormones is the only way to mimic the processes occurring in the human body and provide a support system to our failing hormonal balances as we age or go through significant changes.

Unfortunately, in the pharmaceutical natural hormone market, estrogen and progesterone have been kept apart. The reason? Money.

A patent is only granted to a unique-formula substance, something unavailable in nature. Combining natural estrogen and natural progesterone (instead of a synthetic progesterone) creates a natural combination, which is not patentable. The only way a pharmaceutical company would invest in a combination of hormones would be to make it proprietary, or patentable. And the only way to accomplish this is to introduce a synthetic ingredient. So that's exactly what pharmaceutical companies do. Every combination product that contains natural estradiol is teamed with a synthetic progestin (such as medroxyprogesterone). The problem with this situation is that women who use these products do get the positive effects of natural estradiol, but they also get the potential negative effects of the synthetic progestin.

WHY NATURAL HORMONES IN COMBINATIONS?

After working with hormones for many years and looking at their effects on myself and my patients, I find that I cannot prescribe progesterone alone and expect miraculous recoveries (the only exception is the teenage girl with PMS—she can do great with micronized progesterone alone). This leaves only one way to work with estradiol and progesterone that will provide the results we are looking for—combine the hormones.

The only way to get your hormones combined in one preparation that contains solely natural substances is to have it made to order. This isn't difficult, and it isn't expensive. Combinations of natural hormones mixed to your physician's specifications are made around the country by compounding pharmacies. These pharmacies are replicas of the old-time pharmacies that catered to the individual, preparing each medication specifically for each customer instead of giving out the commercially pre-prepared and packaged drugs that pharmacies now use. These types of pharmacies have been providing the public with compounded natural hormones for years.

So why aren't compounding pharmacies more accessible? Mainly because this is still a cottage industry; most of these pharmacies are individually owned. Their visibility is low with both physicians and consumers. They also lack standardization—because the medications are prepared individually by each pharmacy, what you get at one pharmacy may be different from what you get at another. These factors have kept them off the mainstream radar and prevented natural hormones from getting the recognition and the research funding they need to gain exposure and acceptance.

During one of my lectures to a group of obstetricians and gynecologists, a physician proudly informed me that she was an expert in natural hormones and had prescribed them routinely for more than ten years. She told me her results were remarkable. I was very excited to have her share her wisdom with the rest of the group. I asked her how she dosed the patients and what brands or methods of natural hormones she used.

She announced that every one of her patients received a different amount and combination of hormones. She personally adjusted the doses, often more than once a month. She then added that the situation made her staff and patients crazy. To emphasize her point, she brought her compounding pharmacist along. The pharmacist echoed the doctor's pride in providing individualized services. I asked her how many patients she cared for. She told me she could only treat 250 at a time because the process was so labor intensive.

While using compounding pharmacies to provide women with custom-tailored prescriptions for natural hormones is a great idea, the implementation can become a statistical nightmare. Because it's close to impossible to keep track of the combinations that work for the individual, the data obtained are neither standardized nor user friendly. The information obtained from this type of practice makes it impossible to duplicate or offer standardized guidelines for other physicians to use.

This situation also diminishes the credibility of natural hormones with the conventional medical establishment because it uses antiquated modalities of evaluation and treatment. These are serious problems that leave the public and the medical profession without scientific information appropriate for the twenty-first century.

The only way to advance in the field of natural hormone combining is to standardize preparations and follow the pharmaceutical model for product development and marketing.

PRODUCT STANDARDIZATION

Most compounding pharmacies do not standardize their products. They follow individual physician orders. When a product is standardized, the amount of active hormones is the same in every batch, and rigorous quality assurance processes are followed during the manufacturing or compounding processes. Standardization cannot occur when the products are individually mixed for one patient at a time with varying doses from one prescription to the next. Yet only standardization allows for important statistical data to accumulate in order to evaluate the efficacy and safety of a product. Without standardization, the prescriber and user of the medication have less confidence in what they are really getting.

Because of lack of standardization among compounding pharmacies, the product you get depends on where you get it. If the hormone preparation works, then you're fine. If it doesn't, you and your physician are in a bind. You don't know if the problem is with the preparation, the dose, or the method of delivery (tablets, capsules, creams, drops). Either you give up and assume the hormones don't work, or you have to embark on a search mission that might take months while your symptoms are still there. A standardized product will make your search for the right combination easier and more likely to uncover the source of your problem.

NATURAL HORMONES SHOULD ALLOW YOU TO ADJUST YOUR OWN DOSE (WITH YOUR DOCTOR'S HELP)

The second step in successful treatment with natural hormones is to have the flexibility to self-adjust the doses, with your doctor's supervision, based on how you feel. Natural hormones are not used to treat disease, but rather to treat symptoms of hormone imbalances and to eliminate significant levels of discomfort. It makes sense for the woman who is using them to have the dose tailored to the severity of her symptoms.

Pharmaceuticals manufacture standardized doses for all medications. Physicians have been prescribing medications this way for fifty years. It's a one-size-fits-all mentality. The patient has few choices. If you take the medication as prescribed and it does its job, that's the end of that. If, however, the medication gives you a reaction, makes you partially better, or even makes you sicker, you call your doctor or stop taking it. But stopping may mean you're depriving yourself of a potential cure. The reason you are reacting negatively could be that you aren't getting the right dose. If you, along with your doctor's help, had the ability to adjust your dose, it could solve many of the problems created by commercially available medications.

I certainly don't advocate you do this with every medication; I suggest you work on understanding your body and its reactions to medication and find a physician who is your partner and listens and guides you when prescribing and adjusting medication.

In the case of natural hormones compounded and available by prescription only, the opportunity to obtain standardized dosing with room to individually adjust is available, and I highly recommend considering it.

I find that the best method of administration to accomplish this ideal flexibility and control in dosing is in transdermal cream preparations (meaning you rub them into your skin). After working with natural hormones in all forms, I have found this to be the best blend of conventional medical requirements with patient involvement. Because of the lack of standardization, I spent several years developing standardized formulations for natural hormones, and founded the Natural Hormone Pharmacy in 2002 (see Resources). This is a unique compounding pharmacy exclusively dedicated to standardizing set formulations of estradiol, micronized progesterone, and testosterone in transdermal form.

TAKING A HORMONE HOLIDAY

In the mid-1980s, I spent a few years as an attending physician at St. Cabrini Nursing Home in Dobbs Ferry, New York. It was there that I learned a most important lesson in the art of medicating people.

Most patients on the floor I was responsible for were in their late eighties and early nineties, and at the time, less information was available about the inter-relationship of medications. Many patients were taking as many as twenty medications a day. Diabetes, high blood pressure, heart disease, vascular and mental problems— you name it, it seemed as though the poor old folks received a pill or two for each diagnosis they had. Many were serious pharmaceutical drugs. At the time, I didn't fully appreciate the risks either.

Retrospectively, I wonder how the patients made it through the day so full of medications. I cannot even imagine the number of side effects we must have missed. That was when the head nurse I worked with, Carolyn Doyle, a veteran caregiver, suggested we place the patients on something she called a "drug holiday." After twenty years of experience with the elderly, Carolyn told me in no uncertain terms that the human system needed the weekend off to detoxify from all the pills we were pouring in during the week.

Skeptical at the beginning but respectful of her expertise, I followed her advice. I started a couple of carefully selected patients on the drug holiday; within weeks, they were visibly more alert and their general condition improved. Shortly after we started this program with our selected patients, similar studies in other nursing homes revealed the usefulness of the drug holiday.

So when I started working with hormones, vitamins, and supplements to support hormone balance, I took the concept of drug holiday to my new area of interest.

Thus was born the idea of "hormone holiday." For my patients who have periods, the hormone holiday occurs naturally when they get their period. I advise them to stop taking the hormones while they are bleeding. For patients who have stopped having menstrual cycles, I advise three to four days of hormone, supplement, and vitamin holidays every three to four months.

FALLING OFF THE WAGON AND GETTING BACK ON TRACK

A hormone holiday is good to take when you are feeling fine. Don't take one, however, when you're feeling out of balance. That's when you need to integrate the whole program to get back into balance as fast as possible. When your hot flashes are on the rise, the night sweats and palpitations have made their grand return, your mood is swinging, and your sex drive is dipping, that's when you bring out the big guns—all at once.

You go back on the natural hormones (if you've stopped taking them), you start the hormone-balancing vitamins and supplements, you go on the 30-Day Plan with the diet and exercise, and you do it all starting the same time. Trying one aspect at a time will not work as well as putting all the pieces together.

In the next section of this book, you'll find out what all the pieces are and just how they all work together to help you get healthy, stay healthy, and look and feel terrific.

PART II

THE ESSENTIAL ELEMENTS OF THE 30-DAY PLAN

4

◯

Before You Begin the Program

TAKE CONTROL OF YOUR HEALTH

Before you start the 30-Day Plan, make sure you minimize the possibility that any serious illness may be causing your symptoms. Our health care system is excellent at early diagnosis of disease, so use it to your benefit. No matter how much you hate going to the doctor and how sure you are that the 30-Day Plan is all you need, do get that long-postponed physical, please!

While undergoing your routine physical, though, be aware that the system will often err on the side of overprescribing and overtesting; you want to be cautious, but you don't want to become a professional sick person.

෴

Monica is a lovely forty-four-year-old woman. She raised two children on her own and helps her boyfriend run a diner he owns. Monica developed right-sided abdominal pain radiating to her lower back six months ago. At the same time, her periods became irregular and she started experiencing hot flashes, night sweats, disturbed sleep, and loss of libido. Monica, who had always been active and energetic, found herself almost incapacitated by overwhelming fatigue.

She went to her primary care physician and had a complete physical exam. A full battery of tests including hormones, cholesterol, kidney and liver function tests, ultrasound of her pelvis, and Pap smear, were all normal.

Monica did not feel better, however, so her physician started referring her to specialists. She went to a gynecological oncologist and had a small polyp removed from her vagina, without any improvement in her symptoms.

She saw an endocrinologist, a gastroenterologist, and a neurologist. She had CT scans, MRIs, and colonoscopy, stool, and urine tests. Everything was negative. When I first saw her, she told me her neurologist suspected multiple sclerosis (MS) but needed further testing to establish his presumed diagnosis.

Monica was an emotional wreck. She smoked two packs of cigarettes a day and moved slowly, as though she were made of glass. Her boyfriend was very supportive but was becoming concerned as Monica's life began to center on physicians and testing. She had stopped going to work and was on the brink of tears every time he asked her how she felt.

Fortunately, Monica's story ended well. She realized the answer was not going to be found in continuing the interminable testing the medical profession offered, but rather by taking control of her own life.

Monica came to me after having read *The Hormone Solution*. She suspected that her problems were caused by hormone imbalances. She felt that she would not lose anything by trying the natural hormones, since nothing else she tried had been able to treat or diagnose her accurately.

She asked if I would give her natural hormones and start her on the program while waiting to find out if she had multiple sclerosis. I did. She did not have MS. Monica stopped going for further testing, and within less than thirty days she was back to her normal self.

❧

Monica's story is a perfect example of the dangers of overtesting. Her physicians didn't know what was wrong with her. Instead of admitting they didn't know, they just Ping-Ponged her from specialist to specialist. They never stopped to address her fears and concerns, which were devastating to her.

This doesn't mean you should never go to a doctor or never trust a doctor. It means that you should go prepared with questions you must get answered. Don't take your doctor's advice blindly. Find out exactly why he/she's sending you to a specialist or for a specific test. Ask what the physician will do with the results of the test. How will your treatment course be affected by the test? If something doesn't feel right to you, get another opinion.

Take control of your health! When you go to the doctor, realize it is *you* who must be in charge. You are going to the doctor to get the information you need to improve your well-being. The physician has information and tools to help you, not to scare or confuse you. With this approach, you can and will stay healthy and take advantage of the best the medical profession has to offer.

YOUR MEDICAL EVALUATION

Make an appointment with your gynecologist or internist and get a complete physical examination. Make sure your doctor does a thorough job and becomes involved with you as a whole person. Do not allow anyone to treat you like a body part or an organ. Do not enter a relationship with a physician who treats you with a condescending attitude. The medical evaluation should at a minimum include all the information noted below.

What follows is the intake form I use for my patients. I recommend that you fill it out and offer it to your physician at your next appointment. It should be helpful uncovering issues of hormone imbalances.

PATIENT EVALUATION FORM

Date: _____

Last Name: _____ First Name: _____

Address: _____ Date of Birth _____

Phone: _____ Fax: _____

Allergies: _____

_____

Smoker: Y   N

Alcohol: Y   N

Surgeries: Y   N

Explain: _____

_____

MEDICAL HISTORY

Weight: _____ Height:_____

Still Menstruating: Y   N

Regular: Y   N

Last Menstrual Period: _____

SYMPTOM	YES	NO	AGE STARTED	OCCURENCES
Hot flashes				#/day
Insomnia or sleep disorders				#/day
Night sweats				#/day
Bloating				
Depression				
Weight gain				
Headaches or migraines				
Mood changes				
Anxiety				
Palpitations				

SYMPTOM	YES	NO	AGE STARTED	OCCURENCES
Fatigue				
Irritability				
Vaginal dryness				
Decreased sex drive				
Breast tenderness or soreness				

PAST MEDICAL HISTORY

CONDITIONS	YES	NO	FAMILY MEMBER	SELF
Heart disease				
Phlebitis				
Blood clots				
Bleeding disorder				
Digestive problems				
Infertility				
Osteoporosis				
Arthritis				
Psychiatric Disorders				
Cancer				

List current (or within past 6 weeks) medications
(by prescription or OTC):

_____

_____

_____

_____

_____

_____

_____

_____

MEDICAL TESTING	DATE	NORMAL/ABNORMAL
Complete physical exam		
Pap smear		
Mammography		
Pelvic ultrasound		
Bone density		
General blood tests		
Specific hormone test		
Other		

Since each of us is unique, be aware that my advice here is more general than I would like to be able to offer you, so you must rely on help from your physician to figure out what specific needs you have. Risk factors, family illnesses, genetic problems, and environment-specific issues will affect the type of workup you need. Anything else your physician and you deem important should be done at this time.

Once the results have been reviewed and no medical problem has been discovered, your physician should start you on a balancing regimen of natural hormones. If your physician is uncomfortable or unfamiliar with natural hormones, use the resources at the end of this book to offer him/her help.

Your physician has options on natural hormones. Remember from chapter 3, when we are speaking of natural hormones, we are speaking of only estradiol, estriol, estrone, micronized progesterone, and micronized testosterone. Your physician can choose from compounded preparations of natural hormones or standard prescription-formulary hormones.

If you prefer pharmaceutical natural hormones, they are usually 100 percent reimbursable by insurance, so the cost is low. The problem is that you cannot get both estradiol and micronized progesterone in one preparation, and the dosing of all pharmaceuticals is rigid. Compounded natural hormones are easier to individualize, but they are usually not standardized and the products you get vary with the source. Before deciding which is the best route for you to take, please read the information on natural hormones in chapter 3 and work with your doctor.

Whatever you ultimately decide to use, my general suggestion for dosing based on the average five-foot, four-inch, and 140-pound woman is to start on a prescription of one of the following:

- Estradiol (0.6 mg per day) and micronized progesterone (200 mg per day), either compounded or created by combining preparations available at your local pharmacy (see chapter 3).
- Compounded estradiol (0.6 mg per day) with micronized progesterone (200 mg per day) in transdermal cream form in unit dose.

Do not allow your physician to talk you into synthetic hormone preparations or birth control pills. They will only increase your symptoms and make the transition more difficult to tolerate. They will also interfere with the 30-Day Plan to balance your hormones. If your doctor has not prescribed natural hormones before or used a compounding pharmacy, share the information in this book with him/her so he/she can get you started today.

DON'T LEAVE OUT YOUR
SOCIAL HISTORY

When you're a medical student, your clinical years start with intensive education on how to become a thorough and comprehensive medical interviewer. Without a doubt, a physician who takes a good history is more likely to diagnose your problems correctly and provide better help with your treatment. Part of this initial evaluation involves the Social History, which has more to do with your lifestyle choices (smoking, drinking, drug use) than your medical narrative.

During my medical training, Social History was a limited section of the interview and medical students were not taught to linger on it. History of Present Illness and Past Medical History were considered to be more rewarding in the process of diagnosing and treating an ailment. Not so any longer.

Social History has moved into the limelight. In fact, as medicine is turning from disease treatment to disease prevention, Social History must become the crux of the matter, especially for healthy people looking to stay healthy. Social History now includes evaluation of the patient's lifestyle, diet, exercise regimen, work, and relationships. The list of medications you're asked to provide is no longer limited to those prescribed by a physician; it includes supplements, vitamins, herbs, and anything else you might be taking.

As an informed consumer ultimately responsible for your own health, you must take ownership of your Social History. When you see your practitioners, whether conventional or alternative, give them as much information as you can. Let them know everything you are doing to maintain your health. Don't be intimidated or worried about your clinician's opinion.

If, for instance, you are seeing a conventional physician, share the name of any alternative practitioners involved in your care, how often you see them, and what type of therapies they provide. Don't be afraid that your conventional physician will look down on your using alternative care. He/She desperately needs the alternative therapists' and your help now in the area of disease prevention and evaluation of quality-of-life issues.

Your Social History must become the portion of your care that integrates all the pieces. Do not omit any of the parts if you want to maintain a healthy whole.

DON'T TRY TO BE PERFECT ON THE PROGRAM

If you go into the 30-Day Plan thinking that you must be perfect, you are perfectly wrong. It's not always easy to give up bad habits we've had for a lifetime. Patients ask me this question more often than anything else: "Why do I continue to fall into bad habits?" The answer is simple. We are humans. We are imperfect, and that makes us beautiful and real. We are surrounded by so many options, we don't even know why and how to avoid things that are detrimental to us.

Our culture is about pushing the envelope, seeing how far we can go before we get sick, hurt ourselves, get into trouble. It's all about control; sometimes life is so random we just feel we have to take over our own destinies. But how much control do we really have? We have no input into what is about to happen to us. We can't predict the future, so we try to create it.

Have you every wondered why people become daredevils? Why would folks in their right minds go bungee jumping? Maybe because they're young and believe themselves immortal; maybe because underneath it all, we all know we have no control over what will happen, so we bungee jump!

Well, maybe bungee jumping is an extreme example. For most of us, more reasonable and less daring, pushing the envelope could be something as simple as eating three chocolate chip cookies at 10 P.M. at the age of fifty-four. It will keep us up all night, give us hot flashes and night sweats, and it only means we are trying to prove that we can still do what we did at twenty-two.

Unfortunately, we can't.

We have to understand that everything we do affects the whole of us. When we take a pill—whether a prescription medication, a vitamin, or a natural herbal supplement—or eat a cookie, our whole body is affected by it. If we sleep two hours a night and drink five martinis the evening before, the whole of us is affected. And that includes our relationships. Being honest about our personal life and the relationships we are in is a critical piece to putting the puzzle together. Unless we admit to being totally responsible for being in a bad relationship and developing bad habits, we will never achieve balance in our lives.

5

◯

Feeding Your Hormones:
Your Diet, Your Body, Your Life

If you want to improve your hormone balance, you may have to change the foods you eat. Your diet can single-handedly improve or destroy your hormone balance and, along with it, your well-being.

As a nation, we are obsessed with diets yet grow collectively more overweight. Sixty percent of Americans are obese. Greg Critser's *Fat Land* (Houghton Mifflin Company, 2003), which explores how Americans became so fat, discusses the politics of food. Critser suggests that marketing and greed led to expanding serving sizes and the explosion of the fast-food industry. As a journalist, he even analyzed the health problems created by this situation and the multimillion-dollar industry of treating diseases created by bad foods and bad eating habits that has emerged. The book is a wake-up call to all of us. Diets and medical treatments will not diminish the problem. Changing our eating habits will.

Thirty percent of our children are obese, and the epidemic of type 2 diabetes affects millions. We are obsessed with diets and weight-loss schemes. Girls grow up with ambiguous body images and surrounded by talk about weight control. Although we may hear it a million times, we can't quite grasp that each mouthful we take helps seal our fate in one way or another. From the moment we are born until we take our last breath, we are what we eat.

Yet we insist on turning a blind eye to the connection between how we feel and what we eat. When our hormones are out of balance, we turn to medications, antidepressants, herbal remedies, supplements, vitamins—anything rather than facing an important likely culprit, our diet.

Unfortunately, our dietary habits are hardwired into our subconscious and need to be reprogrammed. The outside world and our American fast-food culture are not going to cooperate in the foreseeable future, so we must take on the responsibility to personally change what we eat.

Suing McDonald's is not the answer. Yes, it would be good if the company listed the ingredients and calorie and fat content of all its menu choices, but would we really care? We can accuse the fast-food industry all we want, analyze why we're fat, find out what is in our food that makes us fat, and read and follow every diet, but ultimately we are totally responsible for the outcome. If we are fat, it is most likely because of four simple facts:

- We eat the wrong things.
- We do not move enough.
- Our hormones are out of balance.
- Our genetics are against us.

So what can we do to improve? First we understand why we are this way.

Our dietary habits, for the most part, are formed at home during our childhood. If you grew up eating junk food, you will likely continue the tradition. You will either follow the same path or make a conscious commitment to change.

I come from Eastern Europe. When I was a child in the 1950s and 1960s, we did not have much food back home in Romania. The concept of freezing foods or adding hormones and preservatives did not exist. Vegetables were available only in season. Fish did not exist as an option, though cod liver oil was a daily torture during long, cold winter months. Sugar, flour, and oil were rationed, and I remember being a small child and waiting on long lines to get our monthly ration. Chocolate was a once-a-year treat, and dairy consisted of the fresh milk, eggs, and cheese a farmer brought to our apartment once a week.

Quite a different picture from the foods my children were raised with in the United States! Even though my childhood eating history is harsh and difficult, my eating habits in Romania turned out to be much healthier and more life sustaining than those I acquired here during my adult life.

Most Americans have no idea which foods are healthy. Often, our most accessible foods have very little to do with good nutrition. The focus in the United States is on presentation, large portion size, and speed of delivery. Our taste buds are corrupted by chemicals and stimulants, our foods chock-full of synthetic hormones. We have been exposed to too much advertising and product placement and too little education about nutrition and diet. We do not make the connections between food and health, food and well-being, food and sustenance.

We do not realize that the American weight problem is directly connected to our constantly fluctuating hormone balance, or that the food we eat is directly responsible for destroying that balance. We will see examples of this connection later in this chapter.

A perfect example of a situation tied into our problematic food intake is the early onset of puberty in our children. Puberty is the time when hormones, dormant since birth, wake up. Girls become women, and boys become men. Puberty is the first step toward fulfilling our mission to reproduce.

In an article published in the journal *Pediatrics* in April 2003, "Percent Body Fat at Age 5 Predicts Earlier Pubertal Development Among Girls at Age 9," researchers found that "Girls with higher percent body fat at 5 years, and girls with higher percent body fat, higher BMI (body mass index) percentile, or larger waist circumferences at 7 years, were more likely to be classified with earlier pubertal development at 9 years." The authors posited several explanations for the link between obesity and early puberty, one of which is that the early onset may be triggered by the excess estrogen produced by greater body fat. They stated, "Research suggests that the central accumulation of body fat has an especially strong influence on levels of estradiol among puberty-aged girls. . . ." The authors concluded that, "The practical implications of these findings emphasize the need for implementation of early prevention and treatment programs for childhood overweight, beginning as early as the preschool period."

I spend my life helping people balance their hormones to feel better, stay younger longer, and avoid chronic illnesses. In this context, I am always taken aback by the negative impact most diets have on hormone balance. Diabetes, hypertension, high cholesterol, arthritis, asthma—all these debilitating, chronic illnesses are worsened and even brought on by the foods we eat, so why do we continue eating them? Why do we continue buying them? Why are we victims?

Knowing that symptoms of hormone imbalance are directly connected to our diets, we can change our eating habits to help balance the hormones and keep us functioning optimally at any age. We may not need to go all-out organic, but we certainly can stop supporting the junk-food industry for starters.

DIET AND HORMONES—
CONNECTING THE DOTS

I first became interested in nutrition during my days as director of the emergency department at Westchester County Medical Center in Valhalla, New York.

You are probably thinking, *What an unlikely place to become interested in nutrition.* At first, I thought so, too. But when I explain why, you'll see that this wasn't such a strange place to start.

I first began to make the diet connections in men in their forties and fifties. They were being brought to the ER with cardiac arrests or life-threatening heart attacks. As we dutifully applied all our emergency skills to their care, I could not help but notice that most of them were overweight, had high blood pressure, and, when asked, admitted to seldom if ever exercising. Many of them were under physicians' care and took medications for their blood pressure problems, diabetes, and other diagnoses they carried. Even so, all the medication did not stop them from getting heart attacks and landing in the emergency room. Their physicians, primarily cardiologists, weren't trained to look at the connections among diet, exercise, and the prevention of heart attacks. The doctors probably made general dietary suggestions, including eating less saturated fats and salt, but didn't offer much specific advice.

When I attempted to suggest we make nutrition part of prevention along with all the medications the patients were already taking, my colleagues did not share my enthusiasm. The party line in those days was to treat disease with either medication or surgery. I was not convinced.

I decided to take a course in nutrition at New York Medical College, where I worked. Even there, little emphasis was given to understanding the missing connection between wellness and diet. There were low-sugar diets for diabetics, low-salt diets for high blood pressure and heart disease, low-fat diets for high cholesterol, low-residue diets for irritable bowels—every diet was after the fact. There were no guidelines available for diets that might prevent illness.

Back in the emergency room, I started my own informal mini survey. I began asking patients about their diets. I heard the most interesting stories. Here are some of them:

ఞ

James, a forty-five-year-old truck driver, was brought to the ER with acute abdominal pain. A large man, he had been on the Atkins diet for two months trying to lose weight in preparation for his daughter's wedding. He had lost thirty pounds—but his gallbladder had been affected. He developed gallstones and in the end needed emergency surgery.

ఞ

Maria, a thirty-two-year-old, followed another popular high-protein diet and ate only shrimp for six weeks. She also restricted her water intake and arrived in the ER in excruciating pain on a Friday at 3 A.M. She said the pain was worse than childbirth. She was passing a kidney stone.

༂

George, a fifty-three-year-old executive with a strong family history of heart disease, was brought into the ER with an acute heart attack. He was thirty pounds overweight, had severe high blood pressure for which he was taking four medications, smoked two packs of cigarettes a day, and drank three martinis every evening. He loved eating his steak and potatoes almost every night. He rarely touched vegetables or fruit.

༂

Jane, a forty-seven-year-old woman, was brought in with heart palpitations at 5 A.M. She also experienced night sweats and insomnia. She tossed and turned every night for six months. The palpitations scared her into coming to the emergency room. She was sure she was having a heart attack. She had eaten a heavy meal with spicy and fried meats and had four glasses of wine and a cup of coffee with her dinner.

༂

I'm not making these stories up. James, Maria, George, and Jane are examples of real patients routinely seen in emergency rooms. Such cases are common, and their frequency has greatly increased over the past fifteen years. Although the people have different names, they mirror the same core fact—you are what you eat. Poor eating habits are what precipitated the problem in each and every one of these cases.

But there is another connection to be made. That is the hormone connection. Let's look at the patient histories with an eye toward hormone balance for a moment.

James was on a high-protein diet. To produce the bile and bile salts he needed to digest this protein, the pancreas, stomach, and liver worked overtime producing increasing levels of digestive enzymes under hormonal direction, changing the consistency of the bile, which in turn led to the development of gallstones. Maria, also on a high-protein fad diet, added insult to injury to her internal balance by not drinking water. In addition to the stress of protein overload, she became dehydrated. This situation directly affected her homeostasis, and to maintain balance her body started to make more hormones designed to preserve the limited amount of water she had in her system. The result was that to hold on to that water, her kidneys concentrated her urine so much that stones were deposited from all the toxins that could no longer be washed out of her system.

George's story is another hormone nightmare. His diet, high in proteins and starches, caused his insulin levels to spike over and over again. Insulin (a hormone) triggers a rise in cortisol, the stress hormone; too much cortisol in the system is dangerous and destructive. Blood vessels get clogged with fatty deposits that block the blood flow to the heart and cause heart attacks.

At the time (eighteen years ago), Jane was a mystery to me. No one knew what was causing her palpitations and night sweats, and no one even suspected that her heavy meal and alcohol consumption had anything to do with her condition. Now that I know more about hormones, however, I believe that Jane was suffering with symptoms of estrogen dominance and decreasing progesterone, exacerbated by her poor eating habits. She is no longer a mystery, and the care she requires should not be difficult to diagnose for any physician. Her symptoms are a direct result of her lifestyle, her hormone imbalances, and menopause.

HORMONE-FRIENDLY FOODS

After twenty-five years of working with patients trying to protect and rebuild health, I have come to believe that average Americans know more about their own personal hormone-friendly foods than most nutritionists. And the reason is simple.

Most nutritionists are tied into particular dietary schools of thought and adhere to their teaching. They are similar to doctors. Conventional physicians will prescribe conventional treatments as they have been taught. Alternative practitioners do the same. Nutritionists are specialists and experts in certain diets and will recommend these diets to their clients. They only give you the knowledge they have. And this knowledge or program may not be the best for your body. If it applies, you do well on the diet; if not, you must continue your search. This is not a criticism, but simply a fact that will actually help you waste less time on diets or programs that are not going to provide you with the help you need. The decision of what program, or in this case what diet, works for you is yours alone.

To be successful, you do not need to become a nutritionist yourself. You do need to become an expert at identifying how you feel, how your body responds and reacts to the foods you eat; then you will always be in the ideal position to determine what food is right for you.

It's difficult, however, when we are given so many conflicting solutions. I have no doubt that you have read every diet book ever written. I don't want you to think about going on "a diet" right now; I want you to look at foods from the standpoint of hormone balance.

To reach that goal, let's do a few things:

• Forget the food pyramid.
• Throw away the diet books.
• Spend time understanding how food affects your hormone balance, not your waistline.

SUGARS

Sugars, also known as carbohydrates, glucose, starches, sweets, and a number of other names, are the mainstay of the Western diet. They include a large number and variety of foods.

Our bodies need sugar because it's the quickest source of fuel for every one of our cells. Our cells need fuel to generate energy and make hormones. Every cell in our bodies has to make energy or else it dies. Regardless of where the cell is located—in the heart, brain, kidney, lung—its survival depends on its ability to make energy.

Sugar is not all bad. As a substrate for cellular energy production, it helps manufacture high-energy molecules. These molecules, called adenosine triphosphate (ATP), are used by the cells to synthesize hormones. This situation makes it very clear that eliminating sugar from your diet altogether will adversely affect your hormones. Eliminating all sugars from your diet is not the goal. But certain types of sugars can be damaging to your system.

The type of sugar you *don't* want is the kind that your body can break down easily. Eating processed, refined sugar—the kind found in such foods as cakes, candies, and most other desserts—results in a rapid rise in your blood sugar. The pancreas responds to this by producing large amounts of insulin (whose job it is to escort sugar to the cells, where it's burned for energy). This is followed by a rapid decrease in sugar and insulin levels, as the sugar, which can't be stored away like fat, is burned up. These fluctuations in your insulin level produce extensive wear and tear on the body.

Sugars that take longer for the body to absorb provide a more even level of sugar to the bloodstream, and therefore a more even level of insulin production. These sugars are found in complex carbohydrates, such as whole grains, vegetables, fruit, beans and peas, and nuts and seeds.

The following foods belong to the category of sugars or carbohydrates that are not desirable:

• **Starches.** Breads and pasta that contain processed white flour, processed white rice, and potatoes.

• **Processed sugars.** Desserts, candy, chocolate, cookies, doughnuts, powdered or refined sugars.

The sugars we should be eating are nonprocessed, raw sugars. They are found in some of the following foods:

• Brown sugar.
• Fruits.
• Vegetables.
• Whole-grain breads and pastas.
• Beans and peas.
• Nuts and seeds.

FATS

Fats are also a great source of energy. Fatty acids, the small molecules that fat is broken down into after it's digested, are building blocks for the manufacture of hormones. Fats are essential to our hormone balance, and understanding the significance of fats and the distinction between good and bad fats is critical to proper nutrition and maintenance of hormone balance.

We have been taught to believe that cholesterol is the worst thing that could happen to us. While scientific data connecting high cholesterol levels with high incidence of heart disease flooded the medical literature in the 1980s, the tides have slowly started turning. It is now generally agreed that cholesterol levels should be maintained below 200 mg/dl in the middle-aged adult. In addition, another side to cholesterol has surfaced.

Cholesterol is the parent of all our hormones. We need cholesterol to make hormones. When low-fat diets became the fad and the Mayo Clinic conducted a ten-year study on males with heart disease who were placed on a zero-fat diet, these men did not have more heart attacks, but they became thin, pale, drawn, and lifeless, without energy or drive. The reason was clear: No fats in the body means no raw materials from which to make hormones. This can lead to rapid aging.

Cholesterol is of utmost importance for the manufacture of estrogen—and it's the body's fat cells that store the estrogen we need when we get older and no longer manufacture it.

We need our cholesterol, even though we need to keep it in check.

Just as we know that there is "good" and "bad" cholesterol, there are also good and bad fats.

In the "bad" category, we have saturated fats, which include animal fats and most whole-dairy-derived fats, as well as the palm, coconut, and partially hydrogenated vegetable oils that are used to make most commercial baked goods. These fats increase the fatty deposits in the blood vessels and interfere with circulation of the blood and oxygen to the brain and other organs. You don't have to give up all fats to be healthy; they're only harmful when saturated fats are the dominant fats consumed.

Other bad fats can be found in hydrogenated oils—oils to which hydrogen has been artificially added at extremely high temperatures to solidify them and give them longer shelf lives. This process, most notably used in making margarine, causes the fat to change its molecular structure into what is called a transfatty acid. These fatty acids have been implicated in increased evidence of heart disease and breast cancer.

The best fats for the body are two groups of fatty acids without which the body cannot function. These are called essential fatty acids (EFAs), and are known as omega-3 and omega-6 fatty acids. Research has shown omega-3 oil to be particularly helpful in reducing heart disease. These oils can be found in most cold-water and deep-ocean fish, such as halibut, cod, salmon, tuna, sardines, and mackerel. Omega-6 oils are found in green leafy vegetables and in flaxseed, safflower, borage, and evening primrose oils.

To stay healthy, you should consume fat in moderation and make sure you eat more good fats than bad.

Good Fats

- Fish oils, also known as omega-3 DHA (docosahexaenoic acid) and EPA (ethyl-eicosapentaenoate).
- Flaxseed oils, also known as omega-6 linoleic and linolenic acids (also found in green leafy vegetables).
- Olive oil—cold pressed and virgin.

Bad Fats

- Transfatty acids (found in margarine).
- Chemically developed synthetic fat substitutes. These can always be identified by their chemical taste; they're found in all preserved foods.

Foods with Fats We Should Use in Moderation

- Bacon.
- Butter.
- Sour cream.
- Fat on meats (steaks, pork chops, skin on poultry, fatty deposits in chicken or beef soups).

Good fats are critical to the maintenance of the integrity of the cell membrane. They help with your moods, stabilize hormone balance, and improve your hair shine, nail strength, and overall cellular function. Balancing your body with the necessary amount of good fats will improve your general health, restore your mood, and give you remarkable energy.

PROTEIN

Protein, which is critical to the production of hormones and the maintenance of hormone balance, comes from two sources: animal and vegetable. Vegetarians often run into problems because they don't get enough protein from vegetable sources alone. All protein sources are good for us; still, our bodies, being of animal origin, desperately need protein in larger quantities and better quality than what we get from vegetable sources. If you're a strict vegetarian, or just trying to get your hormones back in balance, it's wise to add protein concentrates (such as whey or albumin) to your diet to avoid protein deficiency syndromes.

Vegetable Protein Sources

- Beans.
- Nuts.
- Yams.
- Soy.

Animal Protein Sources

- All animal meat, including chicken, turkey, beef, and pork.
- Dairy: milk, cheese, yogurt, buttermilk, eggs, sour cream.

Fish Protein Sources

- All fish meat, such as tuna, salmon, swordfish, and cod.
- All shellfish: lobster, shrimp, clams, mussels, oysters, octopus, scallops, and crabs.

Every one of the above protein sources gets used to make hormones that help maintain muscles, bones, tendons, and cartilage, and help fine-tune the balance in our bodies. Achieving homeostasis is directly contingent upon ingesting enough good-quality protein in our daily diet. It is the quantity of proteins and the balance between the types of proteins that will increase or diminish our chances for success in the maintenance of our hormone balance.

FIBER

Until fifteen years ago, not much was spoken of about fiber in the nutrition field. Fiber arrived on the scene when the connection among sugar, insulin, and weight control was made. Contrary to popular opinion, fiber is not the same as starch—although many starches do contain fiber. In my opinion, fiber is our savior, the foodstuff that protects us from aging. To better understand what this means, let's turn back to hormones for a minute.

As you may remember from chapter 1, insulin is a hormone. It's one of two hormones produced by a thin, long, grape-like gland called the pancreas that is tucked under the left side of your rib cage. Insulin and glucagon (another hormone produced by the pancreas, with the opposite effect on blood sugar from insulin) regulate our blood sugar levels. Insulin pushes blood sugar (glucose) levels down, while glucagon raises them. Insulin and glucagon are the yin and yang of sugar control.

Continuously high sugar levels can lead to diabetes. In diabetes, the balance between insulin and glucagon is off, and the body suffers with heart, kidney, eye, and nervous system problems because the constantly high sugar levels in the bloodstream adversely affect all internal organs.

While insulin helps prevent sugar levels from rising to dangerous levels, it's also a stress hormone. I don't want to beat the "flight or fight" mechanism into the ground, but it is the only mechanism that we humans have to deal with stress. The hormones that are released in times of stress include adrenaline, cortisol, and insulin. The more insulin we make in response to high sugar levels, the more cortisol (the hormone that totally wears down our system) is also produced. Constant spikes of insulin will continuously erode even the strongest of organisms and lead to sickness and aging.

The research involving the connections between insulin and sugar levels is extensive, and for once in the scientific world, the results are consistent. The only way to prevent the damaging effects of insulin imbalance—aging and diabetes—is to keep insulin levels even. That means preventing insulin spikes at all costs.

Fiber helps contain and control these spikes. The discovery that fiber significantly controls the rise and fall of insulin levels has placed it at the top of the list of desirable foods.

How does this work? Most fiber is indigestible. Our bodies cannot break it down; it just floats through our system without being digested or providing the body with many nutrients. Yet it has a very important role. It prevents other foods from being rapidly absorbed into the bloodstream and slows their transformation into sugar. That's how it prevents sudden insulin spikes. So why don't we just eat fiber all the time?

We should, but we can't. There is one limiting factor to the amount of fiber you should eat, a limitation imposed by your stomach and intestines. Because fiber is not digestible, it just lies there. You get bloated from too much fiber and develop intestinal cramps. The amount of fiber you eat should be moderated only by the level of discomfort it provides you. My advice is to eat fiber as much and as often as possible. There is no such thing as too much of it from the hormone balance and well-being standpoints.

Fiber-Rich Foods

- Apples.
- Asparagus.
- Berries.
- Bok choy.
- Bran.
- Broccoli.
- Broccoli rabe.
- Brussels sprouts.
- Cabbage.
- Cauliflower.
- Collard greens.
- Cucumbers.
- Eggplant.
- Grits.
- Kale.
- Lettuce (all types).
- Oats and oatmeal.
- Peas.
- Peppers.
- Radishes.
- Spinach.
- String beans.
- Turnips.
- Watercress.
- Zucchini.

Learn to enjoy fiber and make sure it finds its way to every one of your meals. It is not only a lifesaver, but also a hormone saver.

FOODS THAT CAN EXACERBATE HORMONE PROBLEMS

I have given you brief lists of foods that are good for your hormones; I'll offer menus and suggestions for preparation in later chapters. Once you realize that your hormone balance depends on your food balance, you will see such tremendous improvements in the way you feel that no further convincing will be needed for you to follow the hormone-friendly diet in the 30-Day Plan.

Realistically, though, we live in a world with no commitment to the maintenance of our hormone balance. Our taste buds have long been polluted by marketing and promotional efforts of our so-called modern diets. We tend not to eat the right proteins, fats, and sugars, or to get enough fiber in our diets. We are surrounded by temptation. We are all essentially addicted to many of the very foods that directly destroy our hormone balance and rob us of our youth. Our eating habits encourage wear and tear on our organs and increase the constant stress levels in our lives by leaching the hormones we desperately need from our systems.

This doesn't mean you need to avoid all temptation all the time. You don't have to go to extremes of rigidity to be healthy. In fact, you can get away with a lot. All you need to know is when to stop and where to turn to.

To help, I made a short list of foods with serious potential to throw off your hormone balance and make you feel really crummy. My bet is that you already know what they are. This is only to remind you that when you start feeling badly again, when hot flashes return, or you find yourself waking up at 5 A.M. drenched in a pool of sweat, turn first to these potential monsters in your diet.

If you have indulged too much in the following foods, stop and regroup. Go back on the 30-Day Plan for a month and help your hormones gently slide back into balance and the problems disappear.

The Bad Guys

- Coffee.
- Alcohol.
- Soda (sugar-free and regular).
- Chocolate.
- Ice cream.
- Desserts.
- Too much pasta.
- Too many french fries or potatoes.
- Too much pizza.
- Too much hot and spicy food.
- Eating late at night.
- Not eating enough.
- Too much bread.

That's not so bad, is it?

MONTHLY DIETARY FLUCTUATIONS, CHALLENGES, AND SOLUTIONS

Hormones fluctuate in monthly cycles. So why do we expect to feel the same every time we eat something, regardless of the time of the month? Go back to chapter 1 and remind yourself of which age grouping you belong in to find out how cycles affect your food intakes and hormones.

GROUPS 1, 2, AND 3

Your tolerance for foods is directly tied into the time of the month. Before ovulation—generally the first two weeks of the cycle—you can usually eat pretty much anything and still feel thin, not bloated. You also probably won't crave those midnight snacks. This is because your hormones are in balance. As the estrogen and progesterone balance changes after ovulation and you approach your next menstruation, however, things change on the inside and become visible on the outside.

When pregnancy doesn't occur, estrogen and progesterone start to drop. Unfortunately, they don't do it in synchrony, so often too much estrogen causes you to start craving sweets and salty foods. That's where balancing your hormones with diet, natural hormones, and the 30-Day Plan comes in.

The second half of the cycle is when you want to watch your foods, avoid the "Bad Guys," and follow Weeks 2 and 3 of the 30-Day Plan faithfully. Adding vitamins, supplements, and natural progesterone cream (we'll discuss these later) to the last two weeks of the month helps eliminate the cravings and bring back the hormone balance you need to feel well.

GROUPS 4 AND 5

If you fit into this group, for the most part the cyclic hormonal imbalances you once had are gone. You are now in perpetual hormone imbalance hell—unless you're following the 30-Day Plan.

Take your vitamins and supplements together with the natural hormones as outlined in the 30-Day Plan. The diet becomes a breeze to follow when you have their help. Watch as the problems of weight gain, mood swings, and other symptoms literally vanish.

When you bring in the heavy artillery (natural hormones, supplements, and vitamins), it's easy to eliminate the Bad Guys. All the diets you have tried before are useless in the face of severe hormone imbalance. This is why I start by balancing your hormones first; it's the best way to increase your chances for success.

SEASONAL CHANGES IN HORMONES AND DIET

Have you heard about how seasons affect our moods? You've probably heard about seasonal affective disorder—basically, winter blues. While not everyone becomes clinically depressed when the weather is bad, our hormones are directly affected by seasonal changes. Unfortunately, when we think of mood we're conditioned to look at hormones in the brain (serotonin and dopamine) only. We spend little or no time looking at our hormone balance in general and how estrogens, progesterone, and diet affect our moods and function.

Consider how we address food. What does *comfort food* mean? Food that makes us feel good, right? We eat comfort foods when we are sad, cold, or have the flu. Or sometimes when we are happy or excited. They may include some healthy stuff such as chicken soup, but they are usually starches and processed sweets, like hamburgers, pasta, bread, pizza, french fries, mashed potatoes, chocolate cake, and cookies. But does eating them really make us feel better? Maybe for the moment, but not over time. When you eat these comfort foods, you rapidly increase your blood sugar level, which triggers a spike in your insulin levels, which will make you feel good—temporarily. In the long run, however, the Bad Guys will throw off your hormone balance and wreak havoc within. Insulin spikes followed by rapid drops in your sugar levels increase your appetite, make you feel woozy, and tend to cause you to crave more junk food. Hot flashes, night sweats, depression, weight gain—all the problems will surface shortly after you decide to give into the urge to eat some "comfort foods" when the weather (or life in general) turns bad.

I know that you don't want to give up these foods forever. But are you willing to compromise?

You can start by taking natural hormones, vitamins, and supplements that will help balance the hormones and push the cravings back into their caves while you're waiting for the sun or a better time to return. It might take a few days to get over the cravings, but if you stay consistently on track, you'll feel remarkably better.

WHICH COMES FIRST, THE CRAVING OR THE HORMONE IMBALANCE?

This is the old chicken-or-egg dilemma. My patients often ask me this question once they start connecting hormone changes to their symptoms.

In this case, the answer is simple. The hormone imbalance comes first. But once the cravings show up, the hormone imbalance becomes more difficult to contain and the cravings create a snowball effect that worsens over time. The only viable solution is to take the appearance of cravings as a red flag, a warning about the state of your hormone balance.

AGE-RELATED DIET AND HORMONE CHALLENGES

There is nothing I'd like more than to tell you that I have figured out how at the age of fifty you can eat the junk you ate at twenty-five and feel okay.

I personally have tried every trick to figure out how to do it. More natural hormones, more vitamins and supplements, even more exercise. I failed miserably. The fact is that as we get older, we cannot eat the same things we ate when we were young. It's reality and we must learn to accept it. But accepting it doesn't mean becoming handicapped by our hormone problems. It only means we have to be honest with ourselves.

As we age, we pay for every french fry we eat and martini we drink. And unlike at age twenty, when two days off the bad stuff made you whole again, the recovery at fifty is longer and all too often incomplete. The challenge is to choose special occasions when you should enjoy having that martini, pizza, french fries, or chocolate shake. Sandwich them between good sleep, good exercise, and balanced hormone supplementation, and you should have no problem maintaining a healthy hormone balance.

HOW YOUR METABOLISM AFFECTS YOUR HORMONES

Everyone knows about metabolism, yet few of us understand what it actually does. Metabolism is the balance between the amount of energy our body makes from the foodstuffs we take in, and the amount of energy it uses for activities of daily living. The amount of energy our body uses to live is further broken down into three segments, which are the key to success or failure on the metabolic front. Energy is used to:

- Break down the food we eat into usable fuel for the cells (the breakdown process is called catabolism; the buildup process, anabolism).
- Help us be active and do things like think, run, eat, play, work, and have sex.
- Store complex sugar molecules called glycogen in the liver. (Glycogen is our emergency energy source in case we wind up in a situation without a food source.)

The balance among these activities is our metabolic rate. People with high metabolic rates are often thin and burn up more calories than they store (and everyone hates them). People with slow metabolic rates often feel sluggish and have difficulty shedding those extra ten to fifty pounds regardless of age. They make up 90 percent of the population.

Now here comes the connection: All metabolic activities are controlled by our hormones. As you may remember from chapter 2, our genetics determine much of who we are. Our metabolic tendencies at various ages and stages of life are coded into our genetic material. Although genetics determine our tendencies toward fast or slow metabolisms, we have the ability to change some of our metabolic predispositions. This ability comes from—you guessed it—manipulating our hormone balance, diet, exercise, and lifestyle.

YOUR IDEAL WEIGHT

When I talk about diets in this book, I'm not necessarily talking about losing weight. I am, however, talking about being your ideal weight regardless of your age. If you're looking for your ideal weight, you don't necessarily want to look into an insurance actuarial chart; instead, look at yourself in the mirror and figure out what's right for you.

Unfortunately, in this country we regard "a diet" as the solution to our ever-increasing weight problems. Our obsession with diets and weight loss has caused health problems and confusion, and now that the baby boomers have entered menopause by the millions we are reaping the terrible harvest of a lifetime of dietary abuse we inflicted on our bodies.

The good news is that it isn't too late to change. The bad news is that change cannot be about yet another weight-loss diet. In order to find a nutritional plan that is best for you, you must understand how your body works, how you are hardwired or genetically predetermined, and how your hormones are balanced. Then apply simple basic principles of how various foods affect your hormone balance. The foods and menu suggestions you will find in the 30-Day Plan will help you reach your ideal body weight.

Your ideal body weight is the weight at which you are the most comfortable. You can use charts as guidelines, but remember, no two people are alike, so don't try to fit into someone else's clothes. Don't run to the scale and tell yourself you must lose twenty pounds before you're at your ideal weight. Look at yourself and ask yourself how you feel:

- Are you constantly fatigued?
- Do you have difficulty touching your toes?
- Do you fail to see your toes in the shower?
- Do your clothes fit you too snugly?
- Have you gone up in clothes size consistently over the past ten years?
- Are you having difficulty tying your shoes?

- Do you get winded or out of breath when you go up a flight of stairs?

If you answered yes to any of the above questions, you need to lose weight. But don't embark on a diet to get there. Start the 30-Day Plan and balance your hormones in the process. You will find you'll lose the weight, get back your energy, and look good to boot.

6

◯

Exercise:
Hormonal Benefits of Working Out

The older we get, the bigger couch potatoes we become. We spend more time just watching TV or sitting in front of a computer screen. It seems to be the natural progression of aging. The older we get, the less we move, the more arthritic and stiff our joints become, and the more problematic certain movements are. It's a vicious cycle.

The physical process of slowing down is directly connected to hormone balance. When we are young, our hormones are in balance, we can exercise without trouble, and our movement is free and limber. Our energy is boundless, and we can keep going for long periods of time—and then collapse and sleep for fourteen hours. Our hormones constantly renew and refuel our systems. Even when we're young, however, there are times when our hormones aren't in such perfect balance and we don't feel like exercising or even moving. This example helps make the connection between hormones and movement, exercise, and physical activity even clearer; for instance, how do you feel before you get your period or the first and second day of your period? I remember—and my patients remind me of their similar experiences—barely having the energy to move during those times. Getting out of bed in the morning to go to school or work was an enormous chore. And how about during the first trimester of pregnancy? How often does it seem that just getting up to cross the room is an enormous effort?

Both these examples relate directly to hormone balance. They demonstrate that problems arise when estrogen and progesterone levels are either too low or too high.

Menstruation starts when both estrogen and progesterone are at their lowest levels in the bloodstream. Their disappearance leaves behind exhaustion and depression. During the first trimester of pregnancy when most women complain of extreme fatigue, the amount of estrogen and progesterone manufactured by ovaries and placenta to sustain the fetus are enormous. As a result, the balance among the pituitary, adrenal, and ovarian hormones is changing rapidly. The rapid rise in hormone levels leaves the pregnant woman exhausted.

In time, if we are not pregnant, the cyclic hormone levels are rebuilt and we feel better, at least until ovulation. In pregnancy, by the second trimester our hormones are in better balance and we find our energy levels soaring.

Since hormones influence energy levels, they are also connected to our desire and ability to move, to exercise, and to burn off calories. This connection is present throughout our lives.

As we age and our hormone levels diminish, so do our energy levels. One way we can fight aging is by finding viable ways to avoid becoming stiff, arthritic, and chronically tired.

Just watching your hormones disappear while sitting on the couch will not reverse or halt the aging process. Trying to exercise when hormones are out of balance or missing will not improve your well-being, either; it will strain your system and make you sick as well.

Exercise alone is not the cure-all to everything that some proponents would have you believe. Have you ever noticed what happens to exercise fanatics who work out through thick and thin while ignoring the body's messages to slow down? They often have accidents, look drained, and lose vitality with progressive loss of hormones.

A convincing argument to stay home and watch TV? Not really. The goal is to achieve a balanced exercise life. Easier said than done, you say. Not necessarily so. It's a matter of conditioning. You do integrate brushing your teeth into your life, correct? You don't spend your whole life worrying about cleaning your teeth, and yet for the most part we are all pretty much conditioned to brush our teeth at least twice a day. Why not reach the same level of conditioning with exercise? It certainly is feasible and, above all, rewarding, because you will feel better, and avoid feeling stiff, sore, and old. Movement that maintains flexibility and strength will become routine for you, just like brushing your teeth, taking a shower, or even sitting down and watching TV.

By the time you have completed the 30-Day Plan, exercising—and through it building strength and flexibility—will become part of your daily routine. The results will amaze you, and your well-being, hormone balance, quality of sleep, and overall outlook on life will dramatically improve.

I promise I won't send you to join a gym, force you to become a contortionist, or make you spend a lot of money on exercise equipment or gear. Of course, nor will I stop you if you want to. All I will do is help make physical activity a routine part of your life, help you figure out what activity suits your lifestyle best, and let you experience the internal physical and mental changes that exercise can make in your life.

EXERCISING YOUR HORMONES

Over the last two decades, exercise has become a national craze. Unfortunately, this did not arise from a newfound understanding of the need to use exercise to balance our hormones. The belief that exercise is good for us came more from its impact on metabolic rate and the improvement in physical appearance it offers. We were told that speeding up metabolism would give us higher levels of the feel-good hormones called endorphins and that increasing levels of endorphins would keep us young and healthy. We were told that by increasing metabolic rates, we could lose weight and develop a buff body. The muscular men or women of the 1990s represented the fountain of youth. When we did hear about hormones, it was about treatments with androgens (testosterone) and steroids, which supposedly were the key to buff muscles and youthful looks; these steroids became a "must" for all muscle builders.

But there was another side to the booming hormone and exercise industry.

In the mid-1990s, I started to notice increasing numbers of exhausted patients coming to my office with complaints ranging from sports injuries to frequent colds. These people never got enough rest; they sacrificed sleep for exercise. They pushed themselves to the breaking point just to ensure they got in their daily time at the gym. They exercised at night and in the wee hours of the morning. For many, exercise represented the promise of the perfect body and eternal youth.

Unfortunately, like every promise of perfection, exercise, too, fell short. The only consistent accomplishment of this extreme approach was to increase the incidence of sports injuries, exhaustion, and the inevitable hormone problems. Another lesson to be learned. Exercise works best when it's simply another important part of a consistent program to integrate many areas of life. It cannot be an added stressor; it has to become a routine part of our lives to achieve its real healthy goal of helping balance hormones.

Exercise, physical activity, just moving, are all critical ingredients in the preservation of youth and prevention of disability and chronic illness. In the 30-Day Plan, I will help you formulate the right balance for your exercise program taking into consideration your physical status, your age, your prior exercise experience, and even your interest in exercise.

SOME EXERCISE SUGGESTIONS

There are basically two types of exercise that are important to health: aerobic (or cardio) and weight training.

Exercise is aerobic if it increases your heart rate and makes the heart and lungs work harder to meet the muscles' need for oxygen.

Weight training strengthens the muscles and increases lean muscle mass. It's an example of anaerobic exercise, which does not need extra oxygen. Weight training is especially important as you get older because muscle tissue is seventy times more metabolically active than fat. The more muscle you have, the better you burn fat.

It's difficult, if not irresponsible, to suggest a one-size-fits-all exercise plan. Much depends on your age and physical condition. There are, however, certain guidelines you can follow.

If you're in your teens and early twenties, you should participate in a variety of team sports. Not only does this keep you in great shape, it's great fun. This is the time to make exercise an integral part of your life. If you make being physically active something enjoyable, you're more likely to continue the practice as you get older.

In your late twenties to forties, when you have more work and family responsibilities, it's often more difficult to make time for exercise. But this is a crucial time for physical activity, particularly if you are having children during these years and your hormones are undergoing major changes. This is the time to create a program of exercise that includes aerobics, weight training, and flexibility. Start every day with a ten- to fifteen-minute routine of strength building and stretching. If possible, do three aerobics workouts a week. Swim, play tennis, go hiking or biking. Try to make your socializing include physical activity (go on a bike ride with a friend instead of going out to lunch).

When we get older, the tendency is for inertia to take over. We don't have as much stamina. If you don't continue to build and maintain that stamina, you move less, and as you move less you get weaker. That's why it's so important to begin the exercise habit when you're young and maintain it throughout your life. But be assured, it's never too late to begin an exercise program. The key to exercising when you're older, however, is patience. Older bodies require a significant amount of warm-up time. The start-of-the-day stretching and strength-building time should be increased to twenty minutes. Walk every day. Take Pilates or yoga classes that involve gentle routines with the goal of building your flexibility. Dance. Continue to do the physical exercises you did when you were younger—just be sure to warm up sufficiently before you start, and to cool down afterward.

Each type of exercise addresses different parts of your physical being. The best way to maintain your health with vigor and energy is to address as many parts as possible. It's like owning a car and keeping it in good condition. It's important that you rotate the tires and keep them filled with the proper amount of air—but that doesn't mean you can ignore the engine. Your car will keep getting you where you want to go only if you maintain every part of it.

HORMONES AND INERTIA

The role of inertia in hormone balance is more insidious—and deadly. When you eat the wrong foods, you feel sick. You can choose to continue eating the wrong foods and drinking too much, but eventually your hormone balance will probably become so thrown off that you'll become sick and seek professional help.

Not so with inertia.

Usually, lack of movement doesn't make you feel sick. It's actually easier to sit on a couch and watch TV then to start walking and stretching. But as inertia takes over your life, your hormone balance changes.

The less you move, the less you need your hormones. Your body takes your state of inertia to mean you are hibernating. It's an old mechanism of slowing everything down during periods of minimal movement. Our metabolism slows down, and our hormones follow. An inert person doesn't need the quantity of hormones an active person needs. But if we stay in hormone inertia, we become hormone-drained and age before our time.

No matter how hard I try to balance the hormones of people who lead sedentary lives, I find it impossible to achieve the same positive results I obtain with people who are active.

☙

Geneva was forty-five, single, had no children and worked as a travel agent. She spent her whole day sitting at the desk in front of the computer. At night she went home and ate her dinner in front of the TV set. She loved to socialize with her friends and go to the opera or theater. She hated to exercise but considered herself active and happy with her life. That is, until she started having night sweats and hot flashes, and gained thirty pounds over six months. She became exhausted and could not get any rest.

When I first saw her, she was depressed. She had been placed on natural hormones for her symptoms of menopause by her gynecologist, but the symptoms of hormone imbalance were still present. I advised Geneva on diet and asked her to consider increasing her level of physical activity. She improved her diet but refused to address her sedentary lifestyle. Her condition improved only marginally. She came to see me one more time before seeing a psychiatrist for an antidepressant. I literally begged her to try to increase her exercise for two weeks. She told me she would do this as a favor to me. After much discussion, Geneva agreed to walk for twenty minutes every day and to walk up and down the stairs to her third-floor apartment instead of taking the elevator.

Within ten days, she was feeling 100 percent better and she increased her walking time to forty minutes a day—just because she enjoyed it!

INTEGRATING EXERCISE INTO YOUR LIFE

A few years ago, I was asked to do a consultation on an important businessperson. He was enormously successful and had built a real estate empire that spanned two continents. He was in his early sixties and by all measures his life was a dream come true. He had family and friends at his side and all the toys to enjoy the fruits of his labor. Unfortunately, the man was very unhappy, and he was enormously overweight. He was five feet, seven inches tall and weighed more than four hundred pounds.

He had already seen many experts in the fields of nutrition, endocrinology, and obesity. He had spent time at Duke University, the Mayo Clinic, and at spas in Germany and Switzerland. He had been on virtually every conceivable diet and taken many anti-obesity drugs. At times he lost as much as a hundred pounds, but somehow it all came back with a vengeance when he stopped the particular program. All he saw was an ever-expanding body. He came to see me for testosterone. His endocrinologist had told him that as a last resort, he might try balancing his testosterone levels.

During my couple of hours with him, I inquired into his exercise regimen. He told me he could not walk because he was so over-weight. I was going to start him on hormones and vitamins and supplements, but I knew that this wouldn't be enough. He just weighed too much to lose a great deal of weight without serious physical activity.

At that moment, I felt as sad and defeated as he did. He had looked to me with so much hope, and I knew that without exercise, my program could not help this man.

As a last-ditch effort, I suggested he get a personal trainer and start working out his arms. I figured that this would be easier than walking and would help him get started.

He did, and something wonderful happened. He became a little stronger and realized that even that little bit of movement made him feel better. He continued with the hormones and the personal trainer, but also made another difficult decision: He decided to have gastric bypass surgery to reduce the size of his stomach. Following the procedure, with renewed hope, he increased his exercise regimen.

Over the next year, he lost 120 pounds. He is still seriously over-weight, yet his exercise regimen has now expanded. He walks a quarter mile every day. He also swims and continues the daily exercise routine with the trainer.

If you ask him what he attributes his newfound success to, he doesn't answer, *Stomach stapling*. To everyone's surprise, including his own, his answer is, "Exercise."

7

◊

Supplements:
What You Need for Best Results

Over the past ten years, the over-the-counter supplement business has undergone unprecedented growth—it's now a sixty-five-billion-dollar-a-year industry. The message is clear: Americans want supplements and vitamins. We spend more money on nutraceuticals—vitamins, supplements, and herbals—than on conventional medications. We believe they are safe, help forestall illness, and delay aging. We also believe that because we don't need prescriptions to take them, they give us control over our health and empower us.

A quick look into the history of the nutraceutics industry reveals some interesting facts. Nutraceuticals are an outgrowth of the public dissatisfaction with conventional medical practices; they represent the antithesis of conventional medicine. Many nutraceutics are not approved by the Food and Drug Administration, they are considered foods by governmental agencies (thus perceived safe by the consumer), they are available to anyone without physician supervision, and most physicians know very little about them.

A "focus group" conducted in 1993 by *Prevention Magazine* Health Books discovered that one of the main reasons people were turning to natural options was that they wanted choices. Conventional medicine offers two basic choices: drugs or surgery. When these two options fail, there isn't much left. The movement toward making choices through the use of nutraceutics started in the 1950s when Dr. Linus Pauling, who received the 1954 Nobel Prize for Chemistry, became a vocal proponent of the use of vitamin C. Over the past fifty years, nutraceuticals expanded to an industry that combines three principal elements: vitamins (most of which boast long, established conventional research and track records of safe usage), supplements (with shorter histories and less conventional research behind them, but many with reliable safety records), and herbs (with thousands of years of popular culture usage and little real conventional scientific data behind most of them, little standardization, and unclear safety records).

Nutraceuticals have something to offer for everyone. Most conventional physicians have turned a blind eye and tried to dismiss them for fifty years, yet due to public pressure and consumer trust in them, nutraceuticals can no longer be ignored. Still, there are so many nutraceuticals on the market today—and new ones being touted as the new cure-all every day—that the public is becoming more and more confused. We are in dire need of solid, scientifically based information.

I personally find the glut of vitamins and supplements on the market overwhelming, and the task of choosing which combinations to take daunting. As a conventional physician, I had no definitive source to consult when I became interested in vitamins and supplements in the 1980s. I literally had to conduct my own research, sponsor my own clinical evaluations, and spend time with the gurus of the industry to gain the knowledge and understanding I now possess. I now know a lot about select supplements and vitamins that help improve hormone balance and energy. I do not often recommend herbs because while supplements and vitamins are chemically the same as substances manufactured by our bodies, herbs are foreign to our bodies, much like the drugs we take. Our bodies do not make herbs, and unless herbs have undergone rigid pharmaceutical processes of concentration, purification, and standardization, I personally don't feel confident in prescribing them to my patients, or taking them myself. They, like most drugs, have potential side effects, and because they are not standardized or FDA approved, my confidence in them is low. Vitamins and supplements, although not all FDA approved, are not foreign to our bodies, so they tend to either get absorbed and used as needed by our systems, or pass through to be excreted with our bodily waste products.

After working with vitamins and supplements for close to ten years and seeing the positive results they can offer in the areas of hormone balance and energy production, I have made a list of the ones that I believe, when used correctly, can enhance hormone balance and help keep us energetic and healthy. They have a long track record and solid and extensive scientific data supporting their use. I also find that in the right preparations, created by reliable manufacturers, they are bioavailable (this term refers to the ability of a drug—or in this case, a vitamin or supplement—to enter systemic circulation), and they do work. Here are the supplements I take and recommend to many of my patients, adjusting the dosages depending on their age and medical condition:

- Vitamin C in the morning.
- L-carnitine in the morning.
- Coenzyme Q 10 in the morning.
- Omega-3 DHA in the morning.
- Vitamin B complex in the morning.
- Calcium, magnesium, and zinc in the evening before going to sleep.
- L-glutamine before meals if the patient has sugar cravings.
- Colostrum in the morning and the evening.

Most diet and nutritional gurus would recommend at least three times as many supplements, and most of them would involve combinations of multiple vitamins, supplements, and often herbs. I do not want to discourage you from trying these under the supervision of an expert, but I believe the vitamins and supplements I include in the 30-Day Plan are sufficient to get most people started on the path to hormone balance. Of course, as I mentioned earlier, you should consult with your physician or a nutritional expert before beginning on any supplement program.

I will explain to you why I have chosen these supplements and how their work bolsters our goal of balancing hormones.

As you know from chapter 5, many foods are full of preservatives, hormones, and chemicals. Most of us tend to eat large portions, yet we get little nourishment. In an ideal world, we would return to natural foods—fresh, unpreserved meats and vegetables. And we would follow the seasons and eat what the earth provides. Super-markets would disappear, and along with them frozen and canned foods. The fast-food industry would make a rapid exit. But we don't live in an ideal world, so supplements and vitamins are our advanced society's attempt to correct the imbalances that our bad foods and eating habits have created.

Yet we must watch carefully that we don't create another monster of evolution by overdoing the supplements and vitamins. For this reason, I keep my patients' supplementation down to the most important (in my view) vitamins and supplements.

VITAMIN C

Vitamin C has been studied extensively since the 1940s, and was the first vitamin to receive endorsement by conventional medicine. Dr. Linus Pauling, who brought this vitamin to the attention of the world, believed that it prevented cancer and arthritis and was essentially the fountain of youth. While he may have exaggerated a bit in his enthusiasm, he was not far from the truth. Vitamin C is undisputed, even now more than fifty years later, as the premier antioxidant. Its job is to clean up toxic wastes created by the process of energy production performed by every cell in our body. Subsequently, vitamin C is involved in practically every chemical process in our body. Because it is an integral participant in the chemical reactions that make energy, it is indirectly involved in the manufacturing processes of hormones. Remember, you need energy to make hormones. Vitamin C is involved in the production of blood cells, enhancement of immune function, preservation of cellular integrity, and many other very important life-preserving and anti-aging activities. In short, vitamin C is a superb supplement and true disease preventer. Even if you eat lots of citrus fruits and green vegetables that are abundant in vitamin C, many people can still use a minimum of 500 mg a day as a supplement.

L-CARNITINE

L-carnitine is an amino acid that was originally discovered in the early 1950s in meat. Hence its name—*carnitine*—which means "meat" in Latin. It is not an essential amino acid (part of the elite group of amino acids that make up our genetic material—DNA and RNA) but it is a critical one, an essential building block for proteins and hormones. L-carnitine has been extensively researched for more than forty years. Studies in both the United States and Europe have proven that L-carnitine is an important substrate for hormone production and a critical factor in the process of energy production at the cellular level, in the mitochondria (the energy-making factories in the cells). The scientists at Sigma-Tau, a large pharmaceutical company in Italy, have spent thousands of research hours and millions of dollars studying L-carnitine, and their discoveries have brought remarkable insights into this under-recognized amino acid. From energy production, to moving fatty acids into the mitochondria to help make energy, to its direct involvement in the process of hormone manufacturing, L-carnitine is a very important participant in our well-being. In every cell that contains L-carnitine, hormones are made. I spent three years researching it and using it in my clinical practice, the results of which were published in my book *Natural Energy* (Putnam 1999).

COENZYME Q 10

Coenzyme Q 10 is also known as ubiquinone because it is ubiquitous, meaning it can be found in practically every cell in the human body. It is an enzyme. An enzyme is a facilitator, a helper with chemical processes. Coenzyme Q 10 is an important partner to L-carnitine in the process of energy production at the cellular level. Coenzyme Q 10 is the ultimate antioxidant. A much stronger antioxidant than vitamin E or beta-carotene, co Q 10 is an irreplaceable ingredient in the Krebs Cycle, the energy-making process every cell has to perform to make energy and thus survive. For at least ten years, Karl Folkers, the father of co Q 10, and other highly respected scientists have been lobbying to get coenzyme Q 10 classified as a vitamin. Extensive research on coenzyme Q 10 and the annual publications of the proceedings of the International Coenzyme Q 10 Society have successfully proven direct links between supplementation with coenzyme Q 10 and improvement in cardiac function, decreased severity of congestive heart failure, and diminished need for medication in people with severe heart disease. Information on the cardio-protective action by co Q 10 has increased its use as a supplement in United States, Europe, and Japan by two-hundred-fold in the past five years.

Coenzyme Q 10 has also been associated with improved immune response resulting in heightened protection from infections.

In the process of making hormones, coenzyme Q 10 is important because it helps in the chemical process of high-energy-molecule production in the mitochondria. Energy is then efficiently used to make hormone molecules directly as well as the intermediary to all hormones, cholesterol. In my book *Natural Energy*, I formulated an entire program directed at energy enhancement around my Energy Pack—L-carnitine and coenzyme Q 10. Together with diet, exercise, and lifestyle adjustments, these two miraculous supplements have improved energy and well-being in thousands who are still using them with enthusiasm and great success. Coenzyme Q 10 is found in just about every living cell in plants and animals. So everything we eat contains co Q 10.

Medications used in the treatment of high cholesterol, such as statins, interfere with synthesis of coenzyme Q 10, and many patients on these drugs require supplementation. Coenzyme Q 10 also interferes with radiation therapy, and its use should be discontinued by patients during the active treatment period.

OMEGA-3 FATTY ACIDS

Found originally in fish oil, omega-3 oils are rapidly becoming important components of a comprehensive program of dietary supplementation. The medical profession, with its prejudice against supplements and vitamins, has been slow to endorse omega-3, especially because to the average physician the word *fat* still conjures up visions of arteries clogged with cholesterol plaques. Unfortunately, I believe this archaic mentality has been detrimental to the process of disease prevention of which omega-3 fatty acids are an integral part.

Good fats, described in chapter 5, are essential to our well-being. In the past five years, conventional medical literature has begun to come around to this fact. In December 2002, the *Internal Medicine World Report* newsletter reported on the results of a study that showed "dietary supplementation with ethyl-eicosapentaenoate (EPA), an omega-3 fatty acid found in fish oil, may help relieve symptoms of depression in patients refractory to standard antidepressant medications, according to British researchers."

This finding was based on a study of seventy patients with persistent depression despite ongoing treatment with standard antidepressants. They were randomized to receive one, two, or four grams per day of omega-3 fatty acids, or a placebo, in addition to their unchanged antidepressant medication. After twelve weeks, patients receiving as little as one gram a day of EPA (a type of omega-3 fatty acid) experienced significant improvement in their symptoms.

These data are not unique. Psychiatrists interested in therapies that did not exclusively involve conventional pharmaceutical medications have been using omega-3 fatty acids for more than ten years to help with depression. Many of these doctors report decreases in the patients' requirements for antidepressants and even discontinuation of the medications. Omega-3s offer additional benefits: They do not have any reported side effects (except for a fishy taste in your mouth on occasion), they are another necessary substrate for the production of cholesterol and thus a direct path to improved hormone production, and they maintain and improve cellular membrane integrity (meaning they make our hair shiny, nails stronger, and minds sharper). EPAs are found naturally in many foods, including all fish and seaweed.

VITAMIN B COMPLEX

Replenishing missing stores of vitamin B complex has actually become part of the conventional medicine armamentarium. This supplement contains a combination of vitamins B_1 (thiamine), B_5 (pantothenic acid), B_6 (pyridoxine), and B_{12} (methylcobalamin). B vitamins are found naturally in animal proteins and animal products such as milk, cheese, and eggs.

VITAMIN B_1—THIAMINE

Thiamine is a water-soluble vitamin necessary to help metabolize proteins, carbohydrates, and fats. It is involved in the energy production cycle along with coenzyme Q 10. Its deficiency produces a disease called beriberi or Wernicke-Korsakoff encephalopathy, and was initially discovered during research on nutritional deficiencies associated with alcoholism and other diseases characterized by nutritional starvation such as HIV/AIDS. Vitamin B_1 deficiency is often found in pregnancy, and supplementation is routine in our country. Vitamin B_1 in the B complex preparation helps improve intellectual performance and enhances hormone production and balance.

VITAMIN B_5—PANTOTHENIC ACID

Pantothenic acid is also a water-soluble B vitamin. Its name, derived from the Greek word for "everywhere," suggests the existence of this vitamin in all foodstuffs. The only possible reason for deficiency of this vitamin would be too much processed food and the intake of antibiotics, which routinely rob our systems of nutrients. Vitamin B_5 is also involved in the processes of energy production and hormone formation. Deficiency is associated with fatigue, depression, sleep disturbances, frequent infections, and weakness. Vitamin B_5 is an active participant in the process of hormone synthesis. Because of this significant role, it's often used to treat stress reactions, PMS, and menopausal symptoms, as well as chronic illnesses such as rheumatoid arthritis and even viral hepatitis.

VITAMIN B_6—PYRIDOXINE

This is another water-soluble vitamin whose active form is known as pyridoxal 5'-phosphatase. It is deficient in people with strained and toxic livers. Its most important function is being part of chemical reactions involving amino acids ultimately leading to production of hormones and neurotransmitters. Deficiency in vitamin B_6 is more common than you would expect; it shows up in skin problems such as dermatitis, anemia, tongue irritation, and cracks around the mouth (and you thought they were caused by lack of vitamin C only). Researchers in Japan have conducted animal studies suggesting that vitamin B_6 deficiency interferes with absorption and use of omega-3 fatty acids by the body. Vitamin B_6 is being used in conventional medicine for the treatment of PMS, carpal tunnel syndrome, and to prevent atherosclerosis.

VITAMIN B_{12}

Vitamin B_{12} is water soluble, and is another very important vitamin with multiple conventional medical uses. It is directly involved with the chemical processes that lead to hormone production and the maintenance of their balance and is frequently used in the treatment of male infertility (helps improve sperm quality and motility), sleep disturbances (affects sleep centers in the brain), and immune disorders (helps stimulate immune cell function).

CALCIUM

Calcium is a soft metal, an element (meaning that it's a single molecule—unlike vitamins and supplements, which are made of multiple molecules), and a critical participant in most chemical reactions occurring in our bodies. From being an essential ingredient in keeping our hearts beating regularly, to balancing the production of stomach and pancreatic hormones and enzymes necessary for proper food digestion and absorption, to that continuous source of concern—bone health—calcium is becoming a take-or-age (and become stooped over) supplement. Unfortunately, while everyone advocates calcium supplementation as a panacea, there is a lot of misinformation surrounding this substance.

Osteoporosis, hypertension, and colon cancer have been linked to lack of sufficient calcium. Of course no one has done substantial and reproducible research to find out what adequate calcium intake really means. Anthropological research found that our Paleolithic ancestors, who ate no dairy and very little meat or fish, averaged 1500 mg of calcium a day in their diet. Fast-forward to the present and we find that the average American woman ingests less than 500 mg of calcium a day. Calcium can be found in dairy products such as milk and cheese, and green leafy vegetables like broccoli, spinach, and kale.

Absorption rates of commercially available calcium supplements are poor at best: calcium carbonate 22 percent, calcium citrate 42 percent. Studies show that actual absorption of calcium supplements varies depending on the individual, the chemical makeup of the product, and the production of acid in the stomach. Calcium research in the area of osteoporosis is difficult and frustrating; many calcium trials revealed variation of absorption to be as high as 60 percent among menopausal women studied. Up to 40 percent of the women in the menopausal trials could not stay in calcium balance even though they were given 800 mg daily.

Where does this leave us? The preparation of calcium you take is critical. Most preparations on the market do not provide the proper supplementation of elemental calcium, which is the type of calcium we need. The most readily absorbable preparations are those containing an amino-acid-bound calcium, ideally calcium orotate or calcium citrate/maleate. When bound to an amino acid, calcium has an easier time being absorbed into your cells and providing the element necessary to make bones. However, most preparations with amino-acid-bound calcium are very expensive. The best compromise available is calcium carbonate, which is both absorbable and affordable.

Women with PMS have been found to have low levels of ionized calcium (the form found circulating in the bloodstream, available to the cells) when their estradiol levels rise at midcycle.

A randomized, placebo-controlled, double-blind study of calcium in women with PMS demonstrated that 466 women who received 1200 mg of calcium supplementation a day with moderate to severe symptoms of PMS experienced a 48 percent reduction in symptoms after three months.

MAGNESIUM

Magnesium is another metal (another single molecule), found primarily inside our cells. It is directly involved in hundreds of chemical reactions taking place in our bodies, from maintenance of the immune system to energy production. It is critical for maintaining a healthy system. Women with osteoporosis have been found to have low magnesium levels, and thus supplementation of magnesium alongside calcium is recommended. Magnesium deficiency per se is not usually identified in healthy people. It's found in people suffering with diseases of the small bowel that impair magnesium absorption, in people who take diuretics that flush magnesium from the body, and in people with diabetes where insulin metabolism disturbances directly affect magnesium absorption and use in the body. Magnesium deficiency is also found in people who abuse alcohol, caffeine, and laxatives, because all these conditions affect magnesium absorption and utilization. Magnesium is found naturally in many foods, including whole-grain products, fruits and vegetables, meat, poultry, and fish. It is also found in fats and sweets, such as chocolate.

ZINC

Another metal element, zinc plays an important role in the synthesis of protein, fat, and cholesterol. It also helps with alcohol metabolism, insulin function, and immune protection. It has direct anti-inflammatory action and has been used in conventional medicine in the treatment of chronic diarrhea in malnourished children. Zinc has antioxidant effect and has been linked to involvement in the improvement of hormone balance through its involvement in the regulation of messages derived from the pituitary-hypothalamic axis. As a dietary supplement, zinc has been scientifically proven to increase exercise performance and immune function in the elderly. Zinc has a long track record; documented clinical studies and laboratory experiments prove its effectiveness in the treatment of cold sores, early prevention of viral syndromes, and general immune system stimulation. It can be found in meat, dairy, and whole-grain products.

L-GLUTAMINE

L-glutamine, which is stored primarily in muscle cells, is the most prevalent amino acid in our bloodstream, and is considered a nonessential amino acid like L-carnitine because our cells synthesize it and it does not belong to the group of amino acids that make up our genetic material. In times of metabolic stress, L-glutamine is depleted and supplementation is indicated. L-glutamine is involved in the cleanup of ammonia (a toxic waste product of amino acids, protein, and hormone production), and serves an important function in stabilization of blood sugar levels. L-glutamine prevents insulin spikes through a mechanism of checks and balances of the blood sugar level. Research demonstrates that glutamine supplementation may be beneficial in wound healing, as well as immune enhancement in endurance athletes (through insulin-level stabilization, creating less wear and tear on the system). L-glutamine can be found in beans, fish, meat, and dairy products.

COLOSTRUM

Often called "Mother Nature's perfect combination of immunoglobulins, antibodies, and immune enhancers," colostrum is the first mother's milk. It provides protection to the newborn from viruses, infections, allergens, and toxins. Scientific estimates reveal that colostrum triggers a large number of processes in the newborn that provide lasting benefits—often for a lifetime. As we age, our bodies produce fewer immune factors to fight disease and heal illnesses. Colostrum has been connected with increased ability to protect and enhance immune system reactions and to participate in disease prevention. Bovine colostrum (from cows) is used most often, because it has been proven to contain immune globulins identical to the human immune globulin (which means it is accepted by the human body as its own). In fact, colostrum from cows is even richer than human colostrum in immune factors, especially when it contains the high degree of water solubility from certified grade-A cows. Although this product can be hard to find, the one I prefer is produced by Symbiotics (see Resources).

I advise this basic supplement regimen to help improve my patients' chances of balancing hormones and enhancing the results obtained by combining all parts of the 30-Day Plan.

DR. ERIKA'S ESSENTIAL ELEMENTS SUPPLEMENTS

As you will see in the 30-Day Plan, you can start taking these supplements one by one, until you are taking all of them by the end of the plan. There is another option, and that is to take these supplements in a combination, such as the Essential Elements line I have developed. There are three different combinations, and they are best taken according to your age group.

ESSENTIAL ELEMENTS I (FOR WOMEN YOUNGER THAN 45)

Women at this age are at their peak physical performance level. This combination provides mild supplementation support, especially during times of physical and emotional stress. By checking with your doctor, you can decide when to use this supplement as basic maintenance support and when to double or triple the dose to prevent damage and enhance peak performance. Essential Elements I contains:

- Vitamin C 500 mg
- Folic Acid 800 mcg
- Coenzyme Q 10 60 mg
- Lipoic Acid 50 mg
- Calcium Citrate/Maleate 500 mg
- Magnesium 400 mg
- EPA 450mg/DHA 300 mg
- Iron 30 mg
- B Complex 50 mg
- L-carnitine 500 mg

ESSENTIAL ELEMENTS II (FOR WOMEN 46–60)

Childrearing, career building, marriage, divorce, moves, or just everyday life create hormone changes and continuous wear and tear on a woman's body. Even with great nutrition, exercise, and an ideal lifestyle, a woman's body and mind are subject to the deleterious effects of life. Essential Elements II has been specially formulated for the maintenance of peak performance and the prevention of chronic illness and destructive effects of aging. Essential Elements II contains:

- Colostrum (Bovine, min. 32% IgG) 500 mg
- Lactoferrin 100 mg
- Vitamin C 500 mg

- Coenzyme Q 10 90 mg
- L-carnitine 1000 mg
- Magnesium 400 mg
- Zinc 25 mg
- Calcium Citrate/Maleate 500 mg
- EPA 1000 mg
- B complex 70 mg
- Alpha Lipoic Acid 50 mg

ESSENTIAL ELEMENTS III (FOR WOMEN OVER 60)

The goals here are hormone balance, prevention of chronic illness, and healthy, handicap-free aging. This supplement addresses these key issues, as well as major organ system support. Essential Elements III contains:

- Coenzyme Q 10 100 mg
- L-carnitine 1000 mg
- Alpha Lipoic Acid 100 mg
- Vitamin C 500 mg
- EPA 2000 mg
- Calcium Citrate/Maleate 1000 mg
- Magnesium 400 mg
- Zinc 25 mg
- MSM 100 mg

The Essentials Elements supplements can be obtained at www.drerika.com (see the resources guide at the end of the book). Other brands of supplements combinations are available at many health food stores and vitamin shops. The key is to buy them from legitimate, laboratory-tested sources and in preparations that are bioavailable to your system. Bioavailabilty is critical to success and implies that the substance you have taken will make its way into your system and serve the purpose for which it was taken.

THE GROWTH HORMONE CONTROVERSY

Every time I give a lecture to a mature audience, I get a number of questions about growth hormone—especially when that audience is made up of physicians.

Growth hormone has been used as an anti-aging tool for more than two decades. Taken primarily by the affluent because of its prohibitive cost, growth hormone definitely holds promise in the anti-aging market. Physicians specializing in alternative medicine and anti-aging have created a thriving subculture around growth hormone.

The conventional physician side of me, however, is more than a little skeptical on this topic. I find growth hormone intimidating, if not scary.

Growth hormone is made by the pituitary gland during our early to mid-childhood to help grow the human both physically and mentally. Production of growth hormone declines rapidly in our midteens to early twenties. Adults have ever-dwindling growth hormone levels circulating in the bloodstream.

Anti-aging advocates take the position that growth hormone is actually present well into our middle years and that administering it to older people only replenishes the much-needed substance. They assert that the use of growth hormone is just another hormone supplementation modality to forestall aging and chronic illness.

They are right, to a degree. Growth hormone in injection form has remarkable results. Wrinkles all but disappear, stamina increases multifold, thinking becomes clearer—in a word, you feel and are rejuvenated.

I know what you're thinking—*What's wrong with that? Might growth hormone be the fountain of youth? And if so, why not find the nearest doctor who prescribes it and take it? And why not figure out a way to make it economically feasible for everyone to have access to it?*

Unfortunately, things are little more complicated. Remember that growth hormone diminishes in our bodies in our late teens and early twenties. The human body does not appear to be constructed to make or use growth hormone into its adult years. Data studied and reported are not as widely encouraging on growth hormone as we would like to see.

Should you decide to start taking it in your forties or fifties, your body will begin to think it is growing again. While some parts of your body will be rejuvenated by this event, some may not be. Some people who have taken growth hormone have reported side effects. For instance, in some women, the lining of the uterus started growing again, which led to bleeding. Joint pains were also often encountered due to sudden growth of joint linings. Other side effects included metabolic changes that translated into general bloating and water retention, foggy thinking, and dizziness. Incidents of pituitary enlargement, leading to other unforeseen problems, have also been reported.

While I do not personally prescribe growth hormone, it may be a viable option for some people who are committed to staving off the aging process at all costs. Talk to your doctor before considering taking growth hormone. Be aware that you cannot get meaningful dosages of it without a prescription. Although you may find supplements in drugstores and health food emporiums that claim to contain growth hormone, they don't contain enough of it to make a difference.

8

◯

Journaling Your Hormone Shifts

Now that you've been introduced to the first four essential elements of the 30-Day Plan, you're ready for the last component, which will help you balance not only your hormones but also all the pieces of your life.

You should remember, though, that you don't need to stay on the program all the time. This is not a rigid diet, exercise, and lifestyle program you must follow continuously and exclusively to lose weight, look great, and feel great. It's a program that becomes a lifetime guide for you to pick up anytime you feel things are spinning out of control or you just need a little extra guidance.

We all know why "diets" fail. It's because you're supposed to follow rigid rules that don't leave space for real-life events that make it difficult, if not impossible, for you to stick to the plan. And once you go "off" the diet, and you feel that you've just "blown it," you go back to bad habits.

With the 30-Day Plan, you should feel safe and comfortable enough to leave the program behind when life calls on you to live it. The program is designed to be rational and reasonable; there is no reason to feel guilty if you, like every other human being, are not perfect.

The 30-Day Plan will help you balance your hormones and your life regardless of your age, irrespective of your gender. Men and women of all ages have been following this program for the past five years in my practice, and the results are invariably the same—successful.

To ensure success, you must add this last piece to your program: the journal. You will find it amazing how much better you do with this tool, which allows you to follow your progress, uncover problems, and evaluate areas that need more work. A whole new area of personal awareness will open to you.

At the beginning, nobody likes keeping a journal. It takes time out of our already crowded schedules. It requires commitment and honesty. But it's worth it. We are so busy with our lives working, raising families, going out with our friends, that we never have time to look at ourselves and actually evaluate how different parts of our existence impact the whole. When you become committed to it, you will find your journal a most helpful tool to integrate your life with ease and pleasure.

The journal is a comprehensive diary of your diet, exercise, and lifestyle. I recommend keeping it on a daily basis for a minimum of thirty days. Many of my patients keep it beyond the 30-Day Plan, especially during times of change or stress. It plays a very important role in making a solid connection between cause and effect, and is a useful tool to help you find sources for symptoms of hormone imbalance and life changes that may otherwise elude you.

As you will notice, the journal in this book is more comprehensive than other diaries or journals you may have kept before. That is because most other journals are specifically created to address particular areas of your life. If you are seeing a nutritionist, you are asked to keep a food diary. If you are seeing a psychologist or psychiatrist, you are asked to keep a dream, relationship, or general journal focusing on your emotions. A trainer or physical therapist might ask you to keep a diary of the exercise regimen you are following.

What I'm asking you to do is integrate diet, exercise, lifestyle, relationships, moods, and symptoms—and connect them all to your hormone balance and sense of well-being.

FORMS FOR CHARTING YOUR FLUCTUATIONS, FOODS, AND LIFESTYLE STRESSORS

DAILY JOURNAL

Calendar Day_____

Day of Cycle_____

(Day 1 = Start of Period)

*One chart to be filled out for each day.

DIET

BREAKFAST	Time	Amount	Food Brand
LUNCH	Time	Amount	Food Brand
DINNER	Time	Amount	Food Brand

SNACKS	Time	Amount	Food Brand
LIQUIDS	Type	Amount	

EXERCISE

PHYSICAL ACTIVITIES	Walking	Biking	Swimming	Gym	Pilates	Aerobics	Spinning	Yoga	Elliptical Trainer
AMOUNT OF TIME SPENT									
OTHER									
AMOUNT OF TIME SPENT									

LIFESTYLE

WORK/SCHOOL	Gratifying	Satisfying	Rewarding	Exciting	Stressful	Boring	Terrible	N/A
RELATIONSHIPS	Gratifying	Satisfying	Rewarding	Exciting	Stressful	Boring	Terrible	N/A
MOOD	Good		Indifferent		Bad		Other	
SLEEP (NUMBER OF HOURS)	Continuous		Interrupted					
STRESS LEVEL (RATE 1–5)								
OVERALL RATING OF THE DAY (RATE 1–5)								

1=EXCELLENT

5=POOR

LEARNING TO READ YOUR BODY'S SIGNALS

Marissa, a healthy twenty-five-year-old woman, started having symptoms of hormone imbalance suddenly at the age of twenty-two, shortly after she graduated from college. Her problems involved bloating, mood swings, severe PMS, and menstrual cramps. She reached out for help from experts in the fields of gynecology, internal medicine, and psychiatry. These specialists offered partial solutions in their particular area of expertise. She was placed on antidepressants and birth control pills. She saw a nutritionist, who recommended a gluten-free high-protein diet.

Marissa followed most of her doctors' advice without much success. Then she read *The Hormone Solution* and suspected that her problems might be caused by hormone imbalance. She came to see me looking for a prescription for natural hormones.

After reviewing her social history, general medical history, symptoms, blood tests, and notes from other physicians, I agreed that she needed to have her hormones balanced. In addition, I asked Marissa to keep the journal for a month. I told her I believed my role was to provide her with guidance on putting together the whole picture, not just a prescription for natural hormones. I encouraged her to be as comprehensive and honest as she possibly could when keeping the journal. My help would come from noticing things, little missing links and omissions that only the journal could disclose to me. Then I would point them out to her. In the end, it would be Marissa who would gain the most insight into her own life.

When Marissa returned a month later, her symptoms had improved only slightly. She assured me she was taking the hormone preparations faithfully. Next, I turned to the journal. I was not surprised to see a whole section missing.

The area dealing with work/school was left empty. When I asked Marissa why she hadn't recorded anything in this area, she told me there was nothing worth reporting. So I asked her why. Marissa graduated from college with a degree in art history. Her dream was to become a museum curator. Because of difficulties finding a position in such a highly specialized field, she took a job as a secretary in a liquor distribution company. In her own words, Marissa found her job boring and stressful. But she needed the money, so she felt trapped and disappointed. She did not share her feelings with her family or friends for fear of finding no sympathy.

She was holding all this stress inside, and, unbeknownst to her, her body was reacting through her hormone balance. The fact that she did not record her problems with work in her journal was significant. She had erased that part of her life from her consciousness and thus felt she had nothing to write about. When Marissa and I identified this gaping hole in her perception of her own life, she immediately opened up and addressed the sadness and disappointment she felt about her career. She decided to look for a more rewarding job. Her symptoms eventually improved and disappeared once she dealt with her problems head-on. I no longer treat Marissa with hormones or any other medication.

჻

One of the reasons I ask people to keep a journal is to help raise awareness of parts of their lives to which they do not pay attention. When people don't fill out whole sections in the journal, the blanks tell the story. It is these missing links that, when properly addressed, help put the picture together and integrate the whole person.

Your journal is a key ingredient to your success with the 30-Day Plan. Evaluating your entries on an ongoing basis is critical. The entries will give you insight into your own habits and behaviors you are likely to overlook.

The journal will give you direction and point out areas where improvement is possible and needed. If you have been working too hard and not getting enough rest, if your life is spinning out of control, your journal will point out the problem areas and give you the insights necessary to improve or even eradicate the problem.

LEARNING TO READ YOUR INTERNAL CLOCK

Keeping the journal will help in another area as well: reading your internal clock. We all have an individual internal clock. Some of us are best at working in the mornings; others are night owls. The internal clock determines the physiology of which hormones are released when and how they interact to produce the type of person we are from myriad standpoints. Yet it's almost impossible to learn to follow our internal clocks because most of our lives are spent following external societal and time constraints. For instance, we eat and sleep at times established by our work, school, or play schedules. How many people do you know who follow their internal clock? Very few have the option, and even fewer have the time to find out what their own internal clock is telling them.

Keeping a journal is the best way to become aware of and pay attention to our internal clock. Let's look at an example: Say you work the evening shift at your job. If you are constantly exhausted in the early evening and are full of energy in the early-morning hours, you will find the information reflected in your journal. Then you can understand that you're fighting your own internal clock, and that your hormone imbalances are wreaking havoc in your life. I realize you may not be able to change your job, but the information you now possess will make your life easier through better understanding. If you follow the message sent by your internal clock, your ability to improve your sense of well-being will rise.

If things are getting significantly better, use the journal entries to identify the reasons your progress has been so successful. Notice where you started and analyze the differences between your habits at the beginning of the program and those two, four, or more weeks later.

If your improvement is not as quick or as satisfactory as you expected and you honestly believe your expectations are reasonable, the journal entries will help you find problem areas you may not have addressed yet:

- **Consider your diet.** Have you been adhering to the concept of detoxification, or have you been allowing cigarettes, coffee, soda, or alcohol to ruin all that good work?

- **Scrutinize your exercise program.** Have you been steadily increasing your activity level or did you give up the second you started feeling better?

- **Evaluate your sleep pattern.** Are you getting enough sleep or are your work, family, and/or social life taking priority over your body's need for rest?

- **Assess your hormone regimen.** Did you start feeling better within the first few days of the program but now find your symptoms slowly returning? Are you taking the hormones regularly? Do you need to speak with your doctor about adjusting the dosage? Are you taking the right natural hormones or have you taken a shortcut and accepted synthetics or birth control pills?

- **Review the vitamins and supplements you are taking.** Are you following the regimen correctly or have you already forgotten they were even on the list? It's important to be aware that vitamins and supplements work on subclinical levels. This means we don't experience their results the way we do when we take an aspirin for a headache. It takes time to see their positive effects.

To accomplish everything you set out to do is no small feat, so cut yourself some slack and allow time for improvement. You need to make a commitment to yourself and pay attention to all the details for guaranteed success in this process.

MAKE MODIFICATIONS BASED ON RESULTS

If you feel generally improved and are pleased with the results of your work on the plan, do not change anything. Stay on the program, follow the guidelines, and consult your physician regularly. Your improvement should continue, and you should feel even better in time. You aren't tied into exactly thirty days, of course. This program will work for as long as you stay on it—and you can always return to it.

I often find that once my patients start feeling better, they become greedy. They want to feel even better and they want it faster. I certainly don't blame them. It's only human nature to want things to improve all the time, especially when you've been feeling crummy for a long time. While I totally identify with the goal of continuous improvement, I must also caution you of the importance of remembering where you started.

Most people are quick to forget how uncomfortable and sickly they felt before starting the 30-Day Plan. The second they feel better, their expectation level rises and they want to be twenty again. By all means, let's strive to keep feeling better, but let's not forget how we struggled to find the source of the problem. Let's keep in mind how old and drained we felt when we started, once we no longer feel that way. Let's not overlook the months and years spent on tests and doctors trying to figure out why we felt so badly. And let's be realistic about our true age.

The most difficult part of the 30-Day Plan is keeping reasonable expectations in place. If you are able to maintain reasonable expectations, you can help keep your hormones balanced and feel good as you age.

As you follow the program, you and your physician may have to make modifications. Be assured, however, that in the more than one thousand patients who have participated in the program to date, such changes are usually minimal. More than 75 percent of the time, changes consist of small adjustments in diet, exercise, or lifestyle, yielding phenomenal results.

PART III

DR. ERIKA'S
30-DAY PLAN

9

◯

The Journey Begins:
Days 1–5

Now you know all the key elements that go into this program: natural hormones, diet, exercise, supplements, and journal. Every single one of these elements is essential. They work together. You can achieve some results by improving just one or two of these elements, but if you want to help balance your hormones and achieve total health (and isn't that why you're reading this book?), you need to include all the elements in your new lifestyle.

That doesn't mean you have to change everything at once. There's a reason this is a 30-Day Plan. During the first five days, you'll make small changes, subtract some bad habits, add some good ones. Mostly these days are about mindfulness—about becoming aware of how simple changes can reduce destructive behavior, make you feel significantly better, and set you on the road to a healthier life.

By Day 14, you should notice a major difference. If the program is working for you, your hormones should be in much better balance. Your symptoms should begin to disappear. You should find it easier and easier to follow the program. You should no longer crave every sweet in sight, spend the nights tossing and turning in a pool of sweat, or get up more exhausted than when you went to bed. These significant improvements in your well-being should heighten your commitment to the program as a whole.

By the time you're ready to start this program, you should already have completed the steps outlined in chapter 4. This means that you've already seen your doctor, had a medical evaluation, and discussed the 30-Day Plan with your physician. On Day 1, you will start taking the natural hormones—0.6 mg estradiol and 200 mg micronized progesterone, or a similar combination your doctor has recommended for you, as long as it's all natural, not a synthetic or a combination of natural and synthetic.

As you go through the program, you should constantly refer to previous chapters if you have questions about any of the five elements included. For instance, if I recommend on any day a particular meal that includes salmon, and you hate salmon, simply substitute another healthy protein source. On Day 1, I'll give you specific food suggestions. On days following, I'll give you more options. I don't expect you to follow this plan exactly the way it's written, or to force yourself to eat foods you hate. Follow the program with the goal of making it work best for you.

The Day 1 scenario painted here is for someone who is starting from scratch. If you're already doing more than is required of you at the beginning, don't stop doing it. For instance, the goal is to get you to drink eight glasses of water a day. If you're already doing this, don't go back to one or two glasses because that's what it says here for Day 1. If your diet is good but your exercise is poor, concentrate on building up the exercise portion of the program until, at the end of the thirty days, all the elements are balanced.

Remember, the goal is to get you into total balance. Only then will you enjoy the benefits of putting all the pieces together.

HOW TO FOLLOW THE 30-DAY PLAN

I've laid out the thirty days for you, one by one. Each day is divided into the five elements of the plan: hormones, diet, exercise, supplements, and journal. You may choose to add single supplements one at a time as laid out in the daily plan, or start on Day 1 with the Essential Elements combination for your age group (as described in chapter 7) and continue to take the appropriate choice throughout the thirty days. The groundwork is laid out in Day 1, with new elements being added as the days progress. If nothing new is added or there are no changes, I've simply said "same as Day ___," and you follow the same plan as the day before. Additions and changes on a particular day are marked in bold.

Take it slowly—one day at a time—and enjoy the journey.

DAY 1

NATURAL HORMONES

Estradiol 0.6 mg and micronized progesterone 200 mg per day in divided doses, preferably in cream form. Remember, do not take the hormones while you're having your period. So it's best to start the program at the beginning of a new menstrual cycle.

DIET

- Drink water. Have at least two glasses today. You want to build up to six to eight 8-ounce glasses of water each day. Drink less for a few days before you get your period; otherwise you'll get too bloated.

- Reduce your coffee intake. If you drink three cups a day, have only two. If you drink one, have half a cup.

- Keep track of how much bread you eat each day.

Breakfast

Oz Garcia's Favorite Smoothie

    1 cup orange juice
    5 raspberries
    3 strawberries
    10 blueberries
    ½ scoop Designer-brand Whey Protein Powder
    1 scoop Metagenics-brand UltraClear

Throw into a mixer and blend for 5 seconds. Follow with an 8-ounce glass of water.

1 SERVING

Snacks

Two or three hours after both breakfast and lunch, you must eat a snack. I cannot stress the importance of snacks enough; they are critical to hormone balance because they help you avoid insulin peaks and troughs. Fluctuating insulin levels create wear and tear on the body and are detrimental to your hormone balance. You have the ability to prevent insulin levels from changing rapidly by keeping your blood sugar levels from dropping.

The best way to maintain a stable sugar level is to eat every three hours. As long as blood sugar levels are maintained, insulin will not spike. The foods you choose to accomplish this goal are also critical. You might think that eating sugar would keep your blood sugars from plummeting; this is only partially true, however. Eating sugar will raise your sugar levels and give you a quick energy boost, but it will also trigger a rapid insulin response that produces an insulin level spike. Proteins and fiber are the best foods to eat because they increase sugar levels in the blood gradually and keep them even.

On Day 1, your snack should be:

○ ½ scoop Metagenics UltraClear in 1 glass of orange juice or water. UltraClear is a food-based protein-rich powder designed to help with detoxification. You can find it at most health food stores.

Lunch and Dinner

These two meals are in the same category, because they are interchangeable. If you want to make lunch your large meal of the day, that's fine. If dinner is your main meal preference, that's fine also. What's important is that both meals contain an abundance of healthy protein and fiber.

If you eat pasta, keep track of how many pasta meals you are having in a week. You should reduce this number to one pasta meal a week by Day 21.

○ Before lunch and dinner, drink an eight-ounce glass of water, then wait ten minutes before eating.

○ At least once today, include Erika's Favorite Anytime Salad as part of your meal.

Erika's Favorite Anytime Salad

1 tomato
1 cucumber
½ avocado
1 radish
1–2 cups Boston, red leaf, romaine, or mesclun lettuces
2 tablespoons olive oil
½ tablespoon red wine vinegar
crumbled feta cheese

Toss and salt to taste. You can add olives, corn, hearts of palm, celery, pickles, and any other vegetable your heart desires—the salad will be even more delicious and just as healthy. I like eating this with a slice of toasted multigrain bread. Sometimes I add a can of solid white tuna in water or salmon to the salad, or even leftover chicken, and it becomes a main meal.

1 SERVING

Protein Suggestions for Day 1 Lunch and Dinner

- ¼ pound turkey breast.

- 1 can tuna fish packed in water.

- 1 chicken breast.

- 1 cup tofu.

Vegetable Suggestions for Day 1 Lunch and Dinner

Have any vegetable listed under "Fiber" in chapter 5. Here are some ways to spice them up:

- 1 cup diced white or red cabbage with 3 tablespoons white vinegar and 1 tablespoon olive oil, salted to taste.

- 1 cup steamed broccoli with 1 tablespoon olive oil and a few drops of lemon, salted to taste.

- 1 cup steamed spinach with 1 tablespoon olive oil and a little salt and lemon.

Fruit Suggestions for Day 1

I am not a big advocate of eating fruit by itself, because I find that the sugar fluctuations it induces wreak havoc in our bodies (remember the much-dreaded insulin spike). Used as a dessert substitute or breakfast food in addition to fiber, however, fruit provides occasional satisfaction for the sweet tooth, along with a sudden boost to your energy.

Do not have more than two fruits a day, and do not eat fruit by itself before noon. On Day 1, you may choose from:

- 1 apple.

- 1 apricot.

- 1 banana.

SUPPLEMENTS

Take:

- Vitamin C, 1000 mg per day in the morning.

- Co Q 10, 120 mg per day in the morning.

- L-glutamine, 500 mg half an hour before meals if you have sugar cravings.

EXERCISE

If you're an exercise maniac:

- If you think you cannot live without exercise and feel out of kilter without it, continue your usual exercise routines, only make sure you journal them all carefully this week. Next to the type of exercise you're doing, note the time you spent and how you feel after the particular routine.

If you're a couch potato or used to be a jock but are out of practice:

- If you haven't done any exercises in more than six months, start walking ten minutes a day and journal your reactions.

No matter what level you're at, start Day 1 with the following routine:

- In the morning: Start your day with ten minutes of stretching.
- In the middle of the day: Do five Kegel exercises (tighten your vagina, hold it closed for a count of ten, and breathe).
- After dinner: If you ate out, walk for ten minutes before getting into your car (this is in addition to the ten-minute walk you took earlier). If that's not possible, go home and walk around your house for ten minutes. If you have stairs, walk up and down them for ten minutes.
- If you ate at home, do not sit on the couch as soon as you finish eating. Walk up and down one flight of stairs or around the room ten times.
- Do not engage in serious aerobic or stressful exercises after dinner; you'll release adrenaline and endorphins, which may keep you awake.

DAILY JOURNAL

Calendar Day_____

Day of Cycle_____

(Day 1 = Start of Period)

DIET

BREAKFAST	Time	Amount	Food Brand
LUNCH	Time	Amount	Food Brand
DINNER	Time	Amount	Food Brand
SNACKS	Time	Amount	Food Brand
LIQUIDS	Type	Amount	

EXERCISE

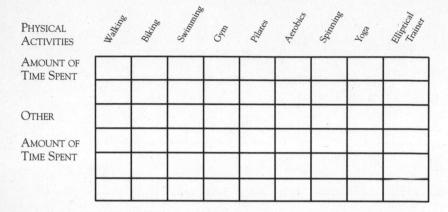

PHYSICAL ACTIVITIES	Walking	Biking	Swimming	Gym	Pilates	Aerobics	Spinning	Yoga	Elliptical Trainer
AMOUNT OF TIME SPENT									
OTHER									
AMOUNT OF TIME SPENT									

LIFESTYLE

WORK/SCHOOL	Gratifying	Satisfying	Rewarding	Exciting	Stressful	Boring	Terrible	N/A
RELATIONSHIPS	Gratifying	Satisfying	Rewarding	Exciting	Stressful	Boring	Terrible	N/A
MOOD	Good		Indifferent		Bad		Other	
SLEEP (NUMBER OF HOURS)	Continuous		Interrupted					
STRESS LEVEL (RATE 1–5)								
OVERALL RATING OF THE DAY								
(RATE 1–5)								

1=EXCELLENT

5=POOR

DAY 2

NATURAL HORMONES

Estradiol 0.6 mg and micronized progesterone 200 mg per day in divided doses, preferably in cream form.

DIET

○ **Drink at least three glasses of water today.**

○ **Reduce your coffee intake to no more than one cup today.**

Breakfast

○ Oz Garcia's Favorite Smoothie (page 140).

Snacks

Include a snack two or three hours after both breakfast and lunch. Have:

○ ½ scoop Metagenics UltraClear in 1 glass of orange juice or water.

Lunch and Dinner

○ Before lunch and dinner, drink an eight-ounce glass of water, and then wait ten minutes before eating.

○ At least once today, include Erika's Favorite Anytime Salad (page 142) as part of your meal.

Protein Suggestions for Day 2 Lunch and Dinner

Same as Day 1.

Vegetable Suggestions for Day 2 Lunch and Dinner

- Same as Day 1.
- 1 cup steamed brussels sprouts with 1 tablespoon olive oil, 1 crushed garlic clove, salt, and pepper.

Fruit Suggestions for Day 2

- Same as Day 1.
- ½ medium cantaloupe.

SUPPLEMENTS

Take:

- Vitamin C, 1000 mg per day in the morning.
- Co Q 10, 120 mg per day in the morning.
- L-glutamine, 500 mg half an hour before meals if you have sugar cravings.

EXERCISE

Same as Day 1.

DAILY JOURNAL

Calendar Day_____

Day of Cycle_____

(Day 1 = Start of Period)

DIET

BREAKFAST	Time	Amount	Food Brand
LUNCH	Time	Amount	Food Brand
DINNER	Time	Amount	Food Brand
SNACKS	Time	Amount	Food Brand
LIQUIDS	Type	Amount	

EXERCISE

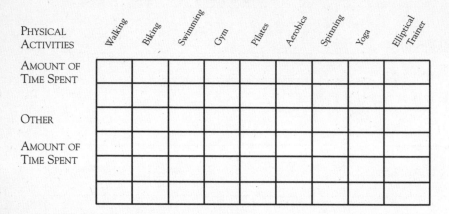

PHYSICAL ACTIVITIES	Walking	Biking	Swimming	Gym	Pilates	Aerobics	Spinning	Yoga	Elliptical Trainer
AMOUNT OF TIME SPENT									
OTHER									
AMOUNT OF TIME SPENT									

LIFESTYLE

WORK/SCHOOL	Gratifying	Satisfying	Rewarding	Exciting	Stressful	Boring	Terrible	N/A
RELATIONSHIPS	Gratifying	Satisfying	Rewarding	Exciting	Stressful	Boring	Terrible	N/A
MOOD	Good		Indifferent		Bad		Other	
SLEEP (NUMBER OF HOURS)	Continuous		Interrupted					
STRESS LEVEL (RATE 1–5)								
OVERALL RATING OF THE DAY (RATE 1–5)								

1=EXCELLENT
5=POOR

DAY 3

NATURAL HORMONES

Same as Day 2.

DIET

- Drink at least three glasses of water today.
- Reduce your coffee intake to no more than one cup today.

Breakfast

- Oz Garcia's Favorite Smoothie (page 140).

Snacks

Same as Day 2.

Lunch and Dinner

- Before lunch and dinner, drink an eight-ounce glass of water, and then wait ten minutes before eating.
- At least once today, include Erika's Favorite Anytime Salad (page 142) as part of your meal.

Protein Suggestions for Day 3 Lunch and Dinner

Same as Day 1.

Vegetable Suggestions for Day 3 Lunch and Dinner

- Same as Day 2.
- **1 cucumber.**

Fruit Suggestions for Day 3

Same as Day 2.

SUPPLEMENTS

Take:

- Vitamin C, 1000 mg per day in the morning.
- Co Q 10, 120 mg per day in the morning.
- L-glutamine, 500 mg half an hour before meals if you have sugar cravings.

EXERCISE

Same as Day 1.

DAILY JOURNAL

Calendar Day_____

Day of Cycle_____

(Day 1 = Start of Period)

DIET

BREAKFAST	Time	Amount	Food Brand
LUNCH	Time	Amount	Food Brand
DINNER	Time	Amount	Food Brand
SNACKS	Time	Amount	Food Brand
LIQUIDS	Type	Amount	

EXERCISE

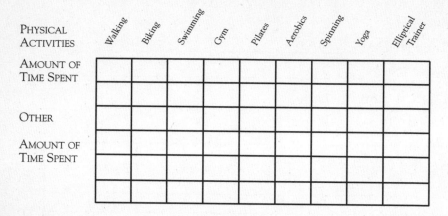

Physical Activities	Walking	Biking	Swimming	Gym	Pilates	Aerobics	Spinning	Yoga	Elliptical Trainer
Amount of Time Spent									
Other									
Amount of Time Spent									

LIFESTYLE

Work/School	Gratifying	Satisfying	Rewarding	Exciting	Stressful	Boring	Terrible	N/A
Relationships	Gratifying	Satisfying	Rewarding	Exciting	Stressful	Boring	Terrible	N/A
Mood	Good		Indifferent		Bad		Other	
Sleep (Number of Hours)	Continuous		Interrupted					
Stress Level (Rate 1–5)								
Overall Rating of the Day (Rate 1–5)								

1=Excellent

5=Poor

DAY 4

NATURAL HORMONES

Same as Day 2.

DIET

- Drink at least four glasses of water today.
- Eliminate coffee.

Breakfast

- Oz Garcia's Favorite Smoothie (page 140).

Snacks

Same as Day 2.

Lunch and Dinner

- Before lunch and dinner, drink an eight-ounce glass of water, and then wait ten minutes before eating.
- At least once today, include Erika's Favorite Anytime Salad (page 142) as part of your meal.

Protein Suggestions for Day 4 Lunch and Dinner

Same as Day 1.

Vegetable Suggestions for Day 4 Lunch and Dinner

Same as Day 3.

Fruit Suggestions for Day 4

Same as Day 2.

SUPPLEMENTS

Take:

- Vitamin C, 1000 mg per day in the morning.
- Co Q 10, 120 mg per day in the morning.
- L-glutamine, 500 mg half an hour before meals if you have sugar cravings.
- **Omega-3 DHA and EPA, 300 mg per day in the morning.**

EXERCISE

Same as Day 1.

DAILY JOURNAL

Calendar Day_____

Day of Cycle_____

(Day 1 = Start of Period)

DIET

BREAKFAST	Time	Amount	Food Brand
LUNCH	Time	Amount	Food Brand
DINNER	Time	Amount	Food Brand
SNACKS	Time	Amount	Food Brand
LIQUIDS	Type	Amount	

EXERCISE

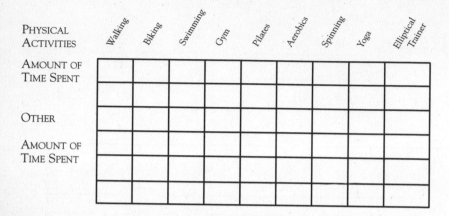

PHYSICAL ACTIVITIES	Walking	Biking	Swimming	Gym	Pilates	Aerobics	Spinning	Yoga	Elliptical Trainer
AMOUNT OF TIME SPENT									
OTHER									
AMOUNT OF TIME SPENT									

LIFESTYLE

WORK/SCHOOL	Gratifying	Satisfying	Rewarding	Exciting	Stressful	Boring	Terrible	N/A
RELATIONSHIPS	Gratifying	Satisfying	Rewarding	Exciting	Stressful	Boring	Terrible	N/A
MOOD	Good		Indifferent		Bad		Other	
SLEEP (NUMBER OF HOURS)	Continuous		Interrupted					
STRESS LEVEL (RATE 1–5)								
OVERALL RATING OF THE DAY								
(RATE 1–5)								

1=EXCELLENT

5=POOR

DAY 5

NATURAL HORMONES

Same as Day 2.

DIET

○ **Drink at least five glasses of water today.**

○ Eliminate coffee.

Breakfast

Have:

○ Oz Garcia's Favorite Smoothie (page 140).

Snacks

Same as Day 2.

Lunch and Dinner

○ Before lunch and dinner, drink an eight-ounce glass of water, and then wait ten minutes before eating.

○ At least once today, include Erika's Favorite Anytime Salad (page 142) as part of your meal.

Protein Suggestions for Day 5 Lunch and Dinner

Same as Day 1.

Vegetable Suggestions for Day 5 Lunch and Dinner

Same as Day 3.

Fruit Suggestions for Day 5

Same as Day 2.

SUPPLEMENTS

Take:

- Vitamin C, 1000 mg per day in the morning.
- Co Q 10, 120 mg per day in the morning.
- L-glutamine, 500 mg half an hour before meals if you have sugar cravings.
- Omega-3 DHA and EPA, 300 mg per day in the morning.

EXERCISE

Same as Day 1.

DAILY JOURNAL

Calendar Day_____

Day of Cycle_____

(Day 1 = Start of Period)

DIET

BREAKFAST	Time	Amount	Food Brand
LUNCH	Time	Amount	Food Brand
DINNER	Time	Amount	Food Brand
SNACKS	Time	Amount	Food Brand
LIQUIDS	Type	Amount	

EXERCISE

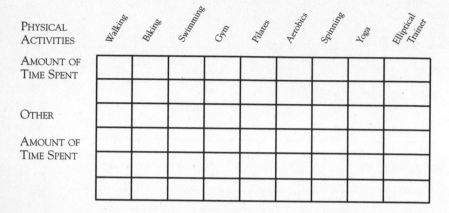

PHYSICAL ACTIVITIES	Walking	Biking	Swimming	Gym	Pilates	Aerobics	Spinning	Yoga	Elliptical Trainer
AMOUNT OF TIME SPENT									
OTHER									
AMOUNT OF TIME SPENT									

LIFESTYLE

WORK/SCHOOL	Gratifying	Satisfying	Rewarding	Exciting	Stressful	Boring	Terrible	N/A
RELATIONSHIPS	Gratifying	Satisfying	Rewarding	Exciting	Stressful	Boring	Terrible	N/A
MOOD	Good		Indifferent		Bad		Other	
SLEEP (NUMBER OF HOURS)	Continuous		Interrupted					
STRESS LEVEL (RATE 1–5)								
OVERALL RATING OF THE DAY								
(RATE 1–5)								

1=EXCELLENT

5=POOR

10

◇

Getting into Gear:
Days 6–10

By now you should be feeling quite a bit better. The goal of this program is to have you improve gradually over a period of thirty days—without adding stress to your life. The plan is not only giving you guidance about what to eat, what supplements to take, and how to exercise, but also training you to pay attention to the way you're living your life.

I don't want you to starve yourself. This is not meant to be a diet to lose weight. You're most likely to lose weight naturally when your hormones are in balance. The mantra for you to remember is that you're doing the best you can with your life and enjoying the results. This is not supposed to be another traumatic experience to prove you are imperfect.

You don't have to be perfect. Make small changes and stick to them, and I promise you'll see the results—and be amazed at how much better you feel.

DAY 6

NATURAL HORMONES

Estradiol 0.6 mg and micronized progesterone 200 mg per day in divided doses, preferably in cream form.

DIET

○ **Drink water. Have at least six glasses today.**

○ **Eliminate coffee.**

Breakfast

Choose either Oz Garcia's Favorite Smoothie (page 140) or a Three-Egg Omelet.

Three-Egg Omelet

1 *whole egg*
2 *egg whites*
1 *teaspoon olive oil*

Beat the egg and egg whites together. Add the olive oil to a pan, pour in the egg mixture, and scramble or prepare an omelet.

1 SERVING

Snacks

Include a snack two or three hours after both breakfast and lunch. For each snack, choose one:

- ½ scoop Metagenics UltraClear in 1 glass of orange juice or water.

- **Protein bar (look for bars that are high in protein and low in carbohydrates and fats).**

Lunch and Dinner

- Before lunch and dinner, drink an eight-ounce glass of water, and then wait ten minutes before eating.

- At least once today, include Erika's Favorite Anytime Salad (page 142) **as either all or part of your meal.**

- **Reduce the number of alcoholic beverages you drink per day by half.**

Protein Suggestions for Day 6 Lunch and Dinner

- ¼ pound turkey breast.

- 1 can tuna fish packed in water.

- 1 chicken breast.

- 1 cup tofu.

Vegetable Suggestions for Day 6 Lunch and Dinner

Have any vegetable listed under "Fiber" in chapter 5. Here are some ways to spice them up:

- 1 cup diced white or red cabbage with 3 tablespoons white vinegar and 1 tablespoon olive oil, salted to taste.

- 1 cup steamed broccoli with 1 tablespoon olive oil and a few drops of lemon, salted to taste.

- 1 cup steamed spinach with 1 tablespoon olive oil and a little salt and lemon.

- 1 cup steamed brussels sprouts with 1 tablespoon olive oil, 1 crushed garlic clove, salt, and pepper.

- **½ head steamed cabbage with 1 tablespoon olive oil, 1 crushed garlic clove, salt, and pepper.**

Fruit Suggestions for Day 6

Do not have more than two fruits a day, and do not eat fruit by itself before noon. Choose from:

- 1 apple.

- 1 apricot.

- 1 banana.

- ½ medium cantaloupe.

- **2 medium slices honeydew melon.**

- **2 cups cherries.**

Supplements

Take:

- Vitamin C, 1000 mg per day in the morning.

- Co Q 10, 120 mg per day in the morning.

- L-glutamine, 500 mg half an hour before meals if you have sugar cravings.

- Omega-3 DHA and EPA, 300 mg per day in the morning.

EXERCISE

- In the morning: Start your day with ten minutes of stretching.

- **Walk for fifteen to twenty minutes today and journal your reactions.**

- **Do twelve crunches: Lie with your back on the floor, your legs bent, and your feet flat on the floor. Clasp your hands behind your head. Do not pull on your neck. Keep your back as flat to the floor as possible. Curl your upper body forward, lifting your shoulders two inches off the ground; hold for five seconds. Don't forget to breathe.**

- In the middle of the day: Do five Kegel exercises (tighten your vagina, hold it closed for a count of ten, and breathe).

- **Sit straight in your chair and suck in your abdominal muscles to the count of twenty. Breathe.**

- After dinner: If you ate out, walk for ten minutes before getting into your car. If that isn't possible, go home and walk around your house for ten minutes. If you have stairs, walk up and down them for ten minutes.

- If you ate at home, do not sit on the couch as soon as you finish eating. Walk up and down one flight of stairs or around the room ten times. Spend ten minutes moving.

- Do not do stressful aerobic exercises after dinner; you'll release adrenaline and endorphins, which will keep you awake and interfere with your sleep quality.

DAILY JOURNAL

Calendar Day_____

Day of Cycle_____

(Day 1 = Start of Period)

DIET

BREAKFAST	Time	Amount	Food Brand
LUNCH	Time	Amount	Food Brand
DINNER	Time	Amount	Food Brand
SNACKS	Time	Amount	Food Brand
LIQUIDS	Type	Amount	

EXERCISE

PHYSICAL ACTIVITIES	Walking	Biking	Swimming	Gym	Pilates	Aerobics	Spinning	Yoga	Elliptical Trainer
AMOUNT OF TIME SPENT									
OTHER									
AMOUNT OF TIME SPENT									

LIFESTYLE

WORK/SCHOOL	Gratifying	Satisfying	Rewarding	Exciting	Stressful	Boring	Terrible	N/A
RELATIONSHIPS	Gratifying	Satisfying	Rewarding	Exciting	Stressful	Boring	Terrible	N/A
MOOD	Good		Indifferent		Bad		Other	
SLEEP (NUMBER OF HOURS)	Continuous		Interrupted					
STRESS LEVEL (RATE 1–5)								
OVERALL RATING OF THE DAY								
(RATE 1–5)								

1=EXCELLENT

5=POOR

A Word about Sleep

Any program designed to improve hormone balance must stress the importance of getting enough sleep. This can be difficult when we lead such busy lives, but it's essential. Scientists have estimated that somewhere between fifty and seventy-five million Americans don't get enough sleep. According to many recent studies, there are a number of reasons for getting a full seven to eight hours of rest every night, including the fact that people who don't get enough sleep tend to eat more. Among other hormonal imbalances worsened by lack of sleep, the hormones that control appetite and weight loss are directly affected.

So pay extra attention to your sleep: the pattern, the amount, and the quality. And record it all in your journal.

DAY 7

NATURAL HORMONES

Same as Day 6.

DIET

○ Drink water. Have at least six glasses today.

○ Eliminate coffee. **Drink one cup of green or regular tea today.**

Breakfast

Have one slice of multigrain toast. In addition, choose from:

○ Oz Garcia's Favorite Smoothie (page 140).

○ Three-Egg Omelet (page 164).

Snacks

Same as Day 6.

Lunch and Dinner

○ Before lunch and dinner, drink an eight-ounce glass of water, and then wait ten minutes before eating.

○ At least once today, include Erika's Favorite Anytime Salad (page 142).

○ Reduce the number of alcoholic beverages you drink per day by half.

Protein Suggestions for Day 7 Lunch and Dinner

○ Same as Day 6.

○ **8 ounces salmon, baked, grilled, or poached.**

Vegetable Suggestions for Day 7 Lunch and Dinner

○ Same as Day 6.

○ **½ head of Boston or 2 cups romaine, red leaf, arugula, or dandelion lettuce, 1 tomato, 1 slice onion (chopped), 1 tablespoon olive oil, 1 tablespoon red wine vinegar, salt and pepper to taste.**

Fruit Suggestions for Day 7

○ Same as Day 6.

○ **1 medium orange.**

○ **2 small tangerines.**

SUPPLEMENTS

Take:

- Vitamin C, 1000 mg per day in the morning.

- Co Q 10, 120 mg per day in the morning.

- L-glutamine, 500 mg half an hour before meals if you have sugar cravings.

- Omega-3 DHA and EPA, 300 mg per day in the morning.

EXERCISE

- Same as Day 6.

DAILY JOURNAL

Calendar Day_____

Day of Cycle_____

(Day 1 = Start of Period)

DIET

BREAKFAST	Time	Amount	Food Brand
LUNCH	Time	Amount	Food Brand
DINNER	Time	Amount	Food Brand
SNACKS	Time	Amount	Food Brand
LIQUIDS	Type	Amount	

EXERCISE

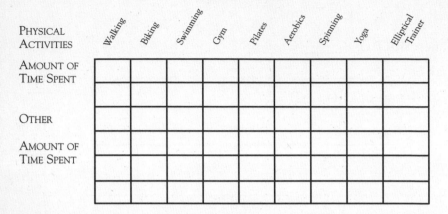

Physical Activities	Walking	Biking	Swimming	Gym	Pilates	Aerobics	Spinning	Yoga	Elliptical Trainer
Amount of Time Spent									
Other									
Amount of Time Spent									

LIFESTYLE

Work/School	Gratifying	Satisfying	Rewarding	Exciting	Stressful	Boring	Terrible	N/A
Relationships	Gratifying	Satisfying	Rewarding	Exciting	Stressful	Boring	Terrible	N/A
Mood	Good		Indifferent		Bad		Other	
Sleep (Number of Hours)	Continuous		Interrupted					
Stress Level (Rate 1–5)								
Overall Rating of the Day								
(Rate 1–5)								

1=Excellent

5=Poor

DAY 8

NATURAL HORMONES

Same as Day 6.

DIET

○ **Drink water. Have at least seven glasses today.**

○ **Drink one cup of green tea, iced tea, or other tea today.**

Breakfast

Same as Day 7.

Snacks

Same as Day 6

Lunch and Dinner

○ Before lunch and dinner, drink an eight-ounce glass of water, and then wait ten minutes before eating.

○ At least once today, include Erika's Favorite Anytime Salad (page 142).

○ **Reduce the number of alcoholic beverages you consume to one glass of wine or one beer a day.**

Protein Suggestions for Day 8 Lunch and Dinner

Same as Day 7.

Vegetable Suggestions for Day 8 Lunch and Dinner

Same as Day 7.

Fruit Suggestions for Day 8

Same as Day 7.

SUPPLEMENTS

Take:

- Vitamin C, 1000 mg per day in the morning.
- Co Q 10, 120 mg per day in the morning.
- L-glutamine, 500 mg half an hour before meals if you have sugar cravings.
- Omega-3 DHA and EPA, 300 mg per day in the morning.
- **Vitamin B complex, 100 mg per day in the morning.**

EXERCISE

Same as Day 6.

DAILY JOURNAL

Calendar Day_____

Day of Cycle_____

(Day 1 = Start of Period)

DIET

BREAKFAST	Time	Amount	Food Brand
LUNCH	Time	Amount	Food Brand
DINNER	Time	Amount	Food Brand
SNACKS	Time	Amount	Food Brand
LIQUIDS	Type	Amount	

EXERCISE

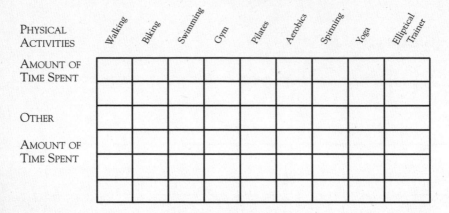

PHYSICAL ACTIVITIES	Walking	Biking	Swimming	Gym	Pilates	Aerobics	Spinning	Yoga	Elliptical Trainer
AMOUNT OF TIME SPENT									
OTHER									
AMOUNT OF TIME SPENT									

LIFESTYLE

WORK/SCHOOL	Gratifying	Satisfying	Rewarding	Exciting	Stressful	Boring	Terrible	N/A
RELATIONSHIPS	Gratifying	Satisfying	Rewarding	Exciting	Stressful	Boring	Terrible	N/A
MOOD	Good		Indifferent		Bad		Other	
SLEEP (NUMBER OF HOURS)	Continuous		Interrupted					
STRESS LEVEL (RATE 1–5)								
OVERALL RATING OF THE DAY								
(RATE 1–5)								

1=EXCELLENT

5=POOR

DAY 9

Natural Hormones

Same as Day 6.

Diet

○ **Drink water. Have at least eight glasses today.**

○ Drink at least one cup of green tea, regular tea, or iced tea today.

Breakfast

Same as Day 7.

Snacks

Same as Day 6.

Lunch and Dinner

○ Before lunch and dinner, drink an eight-ounce glass of water, and then wait ten minutes before eating.

○ At least once today, include Erika's Favorite Anytime Salad (page 142).

Protein Suggestions for Day 9 Lunch and Dinner

Same as Day 7.

Vegetable Suggestions for Day 9 Lunch and Dinner

Same as Day 7.

Fruit Suggestions for Day 9

Same as Day 7.

SUPPLEMENTS

Take:

- Vitamin C, 1000 mg per day in the morning.
- Co Q 10, 120 mg per day in the morning.
- L-glutamine, 500 mg half an hour before meals if you have sugar cravings.
- Omega-3 DHA and EPA, 300 mg per day in the morning.
- Vitamin B complex, 100 mg per day in the morning.

EXERCISE

Same as Day 6.

DAILY JOURNAL

Calendar Day_____

Day of Cycle_____

(Day 1 = Start of Period)

DIET

BREAKFAST	Time	Amount	Food Brand
LUNCH	Time	Amount	Food Brand
DINNER	Time	Amount	Food Brand
SNACKS	Time	Amount	Food Brand
LIQUIDS	Type	Amount	

EXERCISE

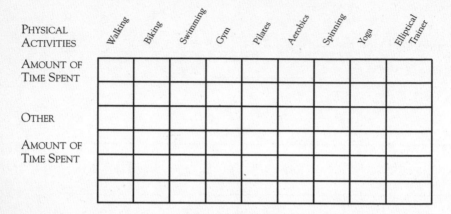

PHYSICAL ACTIVITIES	Walking	Biking	Swimming	Gym	Pilates	Aerobics	Spinning	Yoga	Elliptical Trainer
AMOUNT OF TIME SPENT									
OTHER									
AMOUNT OF TIME SPENT									

LIFESTYLE

WORK/SCHOOL	Gratifying	Satisfying	Rewarding	Exciting	Stressful	Boring	Terrible	N/A
RELATIONSHIPS	Gratifying	Satisfying	Rewarding	Exciting	Stressful	Boring	Terrible	N/A
MOOD	Good		Indifferent		Bad		Other	
SLEEP (NUMBER OF HOURS)	Continuous		Interrupted					
STRESS LEVEL (RATE 1–5)								
OVERALL RATING OF THE DAY								
(RATE 1–5)								

1=EXCELLENT

5=POOR

DAY 10

NATURAL HORMONES

Same as Day 6.

DIET

○ Drink water. Have at least eight glasses today.

Breakfast

Have one slice of multigrain toast and a six-ounce glass of orange or grapefruit juice. In addition, choose from:

○ Oz Garcia's Favorite Smoothie (page 140).

○ Three-Egg Omelet (page 164).

Snacks

Same as Day 6.

Lunch and Dinner

○ Before lunch and dinner, drink an eight-ounce glass of water, and then wait ten minutes before eating.

○ At least once today, include Erika's Favorite Anytime Salad (page 142).

Protein Suggestions for Day 10 Lunch and Dinner

Same as Day 7.

Vegetable Suggestions for Day 10 Lunch and Dinner

○ Same as Day 7.

○ **1 cup steamed beets with salt and pepper and a touch of red wine vinegar.**

Fruit Suggestions for Day 10

○ Same as Day 7.

○ **1 mango.**

SUPPLEMENTS

Take:

○ Vitamin C, 1000 mg per day in the morning.

○ Co Q 10, 120 mg per day in the morning.

○ L-glutamine, 500 mg half an hour before meals if you have sugar cravings.

○ Omega-3 DHA and EPA, 300 mg per day in the morning.

○ Vitamin B complex, 100 mg per day in the morning.

EXERCISE

Same as Day 6.

D A I L Y   J O U R N A L

Calendar Day_____

Day of Cycle_____

(Day 1 = Start of Period)

DIET

BREAKFAST	Time	Amount	Food Brand
LUNCH	Time	Amount	Food Brand
DINNER	Time	Amount	Food Brand
SNACKS	Time	Amount	Food Brand
LIQUIDS	Type	Amount	

EXERCISE

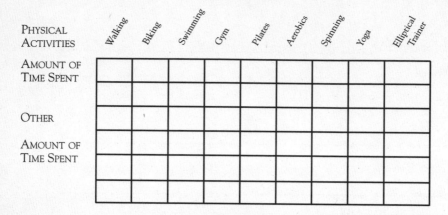

PHYSICAL ACTIVITIES	Walking	Biking	Swimming	Gym	Pilates	Aerobics	Spinning	Yoga	Elliptical Trainer
AMOUNT OF TIME SPENT									
OTHER									
AMOUNT OF TIME SPENT									

LIFESTYLE

WORK/SCHOOL	Gratifying	Satisfying	Rewarding	Exciting	Stressful	Boring	Terrible	N/A
RELATIONSHIPS	Gratifying	Satisfying	Rewarding	Exciting	Stressful	Boring	Terrible	N/A
MOOD	Good		Indifferent		Bad		Other	
SLEEP (NUMBER OF HOURS)	Continuous		Interrupted					
STRESS LEVEL (RATE 1–5)								
OVERALL RATING OF THE DAY								
(RATE 1–5)								

1 = EXCELLENT

5 = POOR

11

Hormone-Friendly Recipes, Part 1

It's often a good idea to keep meals simple for the first thirty days—but that doesn't mean bland or tasteless. In this chapter, you'll find several hormone-balancing recipes you can add to your lunch and dinner selections. They're quick and easy. Be adventurous—if you don't cook, try one and see how you like it. If you're more of a gourmet, look for cookbooks that follow the principles in chapter 5; there are many excellent healthy cookbooks on the market. You might also try some of the more "gourmet" recipes in chapter 16. Also, many supermarkets now have gourmet and/or healthy and organic food sections, where you can pick up ready-made meals. They're perfect for those days when a superbusy schedule has you running ragged with no time to plan or cook.

MY FAVORITE HORMONE-BALANCING RECIPES FOR MEAT, POULTRY, AND FISH

The following are a few of my favorite recipes for entrées that taste good and are extremely easy to prepare, in addition to helping balance your hormones. They're very simple and can be used as guidelines: Improve and expand on them, serving them with the vegetable suggestions in the 30-Day Plan, or others you may enjoy. As long as you follow the basic guidelines of simplicity in preparation, be brave and adapt these foods to your own tastes.

Lemon Chicken Diana

1 chicken breast
1 fresh lemon
salt
pepper

Rub fresh lemon onto the chicken breast; salt and pepper to taste. Place on the grill or barbecue for 20 minutes, turning once.

1 SERVING

Salted Turkey Ozwald

½ turkey breast (1–2 pounds)
rock salt
Lawry's Seasoned Salt

Soak the turkey breast in brine (salt water) overnight. Sprinkle sparingly with Lawry's salt and bake in the oven at 350 degrees for 45 minutes. Serves at least 2 and makes great leftovers for lunch the next day.

2 OR MORE SERVINGS

Salmon Erika Version 1

8-ounce salmon fillet
lemon pepper
garlic lemon spices

Sprinkle the fillet with lemon pepper and garlic lemon spices. Bake in the oven at 350 degrees for 15 minutes. Do not turn.

1 SERVING

Salmon Erika Version 2

8-ounce salmon fillet
5 baby carrots
½ zucchini
3 cherry tomatoes
2 baby yellow potatoes
3 string beans
3 sprigs of parsley
1 teaspoon olive oil

Place the fillet on a sheet of parchment paper. Add the baby carrots, zucchini (sliced), cherry tomatoes, baby yellow potatoes, string beans, parsley, and olive oil. Seal the parchment paper and bake in a 350-degree oven for 20 minutes.

Soy Sauce Salmon Jamie

8-ounce salmon fillet
2 small carrots
1 small celery stalk
1 teaspoon lite soy sauce
½ teaspoon olive oil

Place the salmon fillet on a sheet of parchment paper in a pan. Add the carrots, celery, lite soy sauce, and olive oil; seal the paper. Bake in the oven at 350 degrees for 20 minutes.

1 SERVING

Wasabi Tuna Ken

8-ounce tuna steak
1 teaspoon lite soy sauce
Dab of wasabi

Place the tuna steak on the grill for 10 minutes. Remove, sprinkle with the lite soy sauce and a dab of wasabi, and serve.

1 SERVING

Veggies and Veal Ellen

1 veal chop
3 carrots
2 celery stalks
2 cherry tomatoes
1 small potato
½ teaspoon olive oil
½ cup water or chicken broth

Place the veal chop in a pan with the carrots, celery, cherry tomatoes, potato, olive oil, and water or chicken broth. Bake in a 350-degree oven for 20 minutes.

1 SERVING

Even in the summer or warmer weather, soup is a great food—it's an excellent source of protein and vegetables, and is easy to make and keep. The following is my mother's recipe for chicken soup. It comes from Romania with love and I hope you try it and enjoy it.

Mom's Romanian Chicken Soup

1 chicken
1 parsnip
4 carrots
1 bunch Italian parsley
1 onion
3 celery stalks
1 round large white radish
½ bunch dill
salt to taste

After cleaning all the ingredients, place them together in a large stockpot; fill the pot with water to cover. When the water starts to boil, remove the scum. Cover the pot and simmer for 2 hours or until the chicken meat is easily removed from the bone; discard bones and skin and return meat to the pot. Add some boiled angel-hair or fideos pasta. Then enjoy!

4–6 SERVINGS

12

❑

Moving Up to Speed:
Days 11–15

Have you noticed any changes in the last ten days? Have you made any connections between changing your habits and how you're feeling now? Are you eating any differently? Moving more? Keeping track of changes in your symptoms and moods as the plan progresses?

By the time you finish this chapter, you should be feeling quite a lot better. You're taking the hormones, you're eliminating foods that exacerbate your symptoms, you're taking important supplements. You're probably much less of a couch potato than you used to be just two weeks ago. You're well on your way to integrating all aspects of your life into a fitter, healthier, more balanced you.

Keep it going, even if you're not perfect. Especially if you're not perfect. The smallest of changes will be good for you in the long run. Even if you implement only 50 percent of the changes I've recommended, you should feel better than before. Give the program a chance to work, and you'll be amazed at the difference.

DAY 11

Natural Hormones

Estradiol 0.6 mg and micronized progesterone 200 mg per day in divided doses, preferably in cream form.

Diet

○ Drink water. Have at least eight glasses today.

Breakfast

Have one slice of multigrain toast and a six-ounce glass of orange or grapefruit juice. In addition, choose from:

○ Oz Garcia's Favorite Smoothie (page 140).

○ Three-Egg Omelet (page 164).

○ **Three-Egg Vegetable Omelet (follow the recipe on page 164, but add 1 cup of your favorite vegetables: steamed spinach, broccoli, mushrooms, peppers, or onions).**

○ **1 cup oatmeal in ½ cup skimmed milk, rice milk, or soy milk.**

Snacks

Include a snack two or three hours after both breakfast and lunch. For each snack, choose one:

○ ½ scoop Metagenics UltraClear in 1 glass of orange juice or water.

○ Protein bar.

○ **Designer Whey Protein drink.**

○ **1 apple with 2 slices rye melba toast.**

Lunch and Dinner

○ Before lunch and dinner, drink an eight-ounce glass of water, and then wait ten minutes before eating.

○ At least once today, include Erika's Favorite Anytime Salad (page 142).

○ **No alcoholic beverages.**

○ **Reduce the number of sodas you drink (diet or regular) by half.**

○ **Reduce the amount of bread and potatoes you eat by half.**

Protein Suggestions for Day 11 Lunch and Dinner

○ ¼ pound turkey breast.

○ 1 can tuna fish packed in water.

○ 1 chicken breast.

○ 1 cup tofu.

○ 8 ounces salmon, baked, grilled, or poached.

○ **8–10 pieces of sushi.**

Vegetable Suggestions for Day 11 Lunch and Dinner

Have any vegetable listed under "Fiber" in chapter 5. Here are some ways to spice them up:

- 1 cup diced white or red cabbage with 3 tablespoons white vinegar and 1 tablespoon olive oil, salted to taste.

- 1 cup steamed broccoli with 1 tablespoon olive oil and a few drops of lemon, salted to taste.

- 1 cup steamed spinach with 1 tablespoon olive oil and a little salt and lemon.

- 1 cup steamed brussels sprouts with 1 tablespoon olive oil, 1 crushed garlic clove, salt, and pepper.

- ½ head steamed cabbage with 1 tablespoon olive oil, 1 crushed garlic clove, salt, and pepper.

- ½ head Boston or 2 cups romaine, red leaf, arugula, or dandelion lettuce, 1 tomato, 1 slice onion (chopped), 1 tablespoon olive oil, 1 tablespoon balsamic vinegar, salt and pepper to taste.

- **1 cup green beans steamed with 1 cup tomato sauce, ¼ teaspoon oregano, ¼ teaspoon fresh chopped dill, 1 tablespoon olive oil, 1 crushed small garlic clove, and ½ onion (diced).**

Fruit Suggestions for Day 11

Do not have more than two fruits a day, and do not eat fruit by itself before noon. Choose from:

- 1 apple.

- 1 apricot.

- 1 banana.

- ½ medium cantaloupe.

- 2 medium slices honeydew melon.

- 2 cups cherries.

- 1 medium orange.

- 2 small tangerines.
- 1 mango.
- **1 peach.**
- **1 medium pear.**

SUPPLEMENTS

Take:

- Vitamin C, 1000 mg per day in the morning.
- Co Q 10, 120 mg per day in the morning.
- Omega-3 DHA and EPA, 300 mg per day in the morning.
- Vitamin B complex, 100 mg per day in the morning.
- L-carnitine, 500 mg per day in the morning.

At this point, you should be taking a combination supplement that includes the above supplements. I recommend **Dr. Erika's Essential Elements**, but you can use other reputable brands as well.

EXERCISE

- In the morning: Start your day with ten minutes of stretching.
- Walk for twenty minutes today and journal your reactions.
- Do twelve crunches: Lie with your back on the floor, your legs bent, and your feet flat on the floor. Clasp your hands behind your head. Do not pull on your neck. Keep your back as flat to the floor as possible. Curl your upper body forward, lifting your shoulder blades two inches off the ground; hold for five seconds. Don't forget to breathe.

○ Do twelve side bends: Begin by standing up straight. Drop your head to the left. Once you feel a stretch in your neck, gently slide your left hand down your leg toward the floor. Breathe. You should feel the stretch in your right side. Avoid pulling sensations in your neck. Hold this position and slowly count to five. Slowly roll back up. Repeat on the right side.

○ In the middle of the day: **Do ten Kegel exercises** (tighten your vagina, hold it closed for a count of ten, and breathe).

○ Sit straight in your chair and suck in your abdominal muscles to the count of twenty. Breathe.

○ While sitting, tighten your butt, count to ten, breathe, release. Repeat ten times. Do this exercise after breakfast, lunch, and dinner.

○ Include some aerobic exercises in your routine. Refer to chapter 6 to determine which ones are appropriate for your age group. If you haven't exercised in a while, start slowly and gently. Many gyms now offer nonimpact aerobic classes, which are easier on older joints.

○ After dinner: If you ate out, walk for fifteen minutes before getting into your car. If that's not possible, go home and walk around your house for fifteen minutes. If you have stairs, walk up and down them for fifteen minutes.

○ If you ate at home, do not go sit on the couch as soon as you finish eating. Walk up and down two flights of stairs or around the room twenty times.

○ Do not do serious aerobic or stressful exercises after dinner; you'll release adrenaline and endorphins, which will keep you awake.

DAILY JOURNAL

Calendar Day_____

Day of Cycle_____

(Day 1 = Start of Period)

DIET

BREAKFAST	Time	Amount	Food Brand
LUNCH	Time	Amount	Food Brand
DINNER	Time	Amount	Food Brand
SNACKS	Time	Amount	Food Brand
LIQUIDS	Type	Amount	

EXERCISE

PHYSICAL ACTIVITIES	Walking	Biking	Swimming	Gym	Pilates	Aerobics	Spinning	Yoga	Elliptical Trainer
AMOUNT OF TIME SPENT									
OTHER									
AMOUNT OF TIME SPENT									

LIFESTYLE

WORK/SCHOOL	Gratifying	Satisfying	Rewarding	Exciting	Stressful	Boring	Terrible	N/A
RELATIONSHIPS	Gratifying	Satisfying	Rewarding	Exciting	Stressful	Boring	Terrible	N/A
MOOD	Good		Indifferent		Bad		Other	
SLEEP (NUMBER OF HOURS)	Continuous		Interrupted					
STRESS LEVEL (RATE 1–5)								

OVERALL RATING OF THE DAY								
(RATE 1–5)								

1=EXCELLENT

5=POOR

DAY 12

NATURAL HORMONES

Same as Day 11.

DIET

- Drink water. Have at least eight glasses today.
- Drink one cup of green tea.

Breakfast

Same as Day 11.

Snacks

Same as Day 11.

Lunch and Dinner

- Before lunch and dinner, drink an eight-ounce glass of water, and then wait ten minutes before eating.
- At least once today, include Erika's Favorite Anytime Salad (page 142).
- No alcoholic beverages.
- Reduce the number of sodas you drink (diet or regular) by half.
- Reduce the amount of bread and potatoes you eat by half.

Protein Suggestions for Day 12 Lunch and Dinner

Same as Day 11.

Vegetable Suggestions for Day 12 Lunch and Dinner

Same as Day 11.

Fruit Suggestions for Day 12

Same as Day 11.

SUPPLEMENTS

Take:

- Vitamin C, 1000 mg per day in the morning.
- Co Q 10, 120 mg per day in the morning.
- Omega-3 DHA and EPA, 300 mg in the morning **and again at 4 P.M.**
- Vitamin B complex, 100 mg per day in the morning.
- L-carnitine, 500 mg in the morning **and 500 mg at 4 P.M.**

EXERCISE

Same as Day 11.

DAILY JOURNAL

Calendar Day_____

Day of Cycle_____

(Day 1 = Start of Period)

DIET

BREAKFAST	Time	Amount	Food Brand

LUNCH	Time	Amount	Food Brand

DINNER	Time	Amount	Food Brand

SNACKS	Time	Amount	Food Brand

LIQUIDS	Type	Amount	

EXERCISE

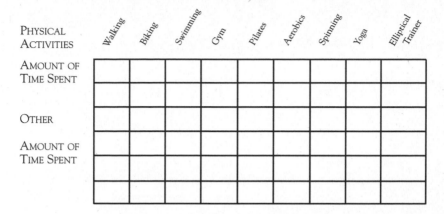

Physical Activities	Walking	Biking	Swimming	Gym	Pilates	Aerobics	Spinning	Yoga	Elliptical Trainer
Amount of Time Spent									
Other									
Amount of Time Spent									

LIFESTYLE

Work/School	Gratifying	Satisfying	Rewarding	Exciting	Stressful	Boring	Terrible	N/A
Relationships	Gratifying	Satisfying	Rewarding	Exciting	Stressful	Boring	Terrible	N/A
Mood	Good		Indifferent		Bad		Other	
Sleep (Number of Hours)	Continuous		Interrupted					
Stress Level (Rate 1–5)								
Overall Rating of the Day								
(Rate 1–5)								

1=Excellent

5=Poor

DAY 13

NATURAL HORMONES

Same as Day 11.

DIET

○ Drink water. Have at least eight glasses today.

○ Drink one cup of green tea.

Breakfast

Same as Day 11.

Snacks

Same as Day 11.

Lunch and Dinner

○ Before lunch and dinner, drink an eight-ounce glass of water, and then wait ten minutes before eating.

○ At least once today, include Erika's Favorite Anytime Salad (page 142).

○ No alcoholic beverages.

○ Reduce the number of sodas you drink (diet or regular) by half.

○ Reduce the amount of bread and potatoes you eat by half.

Protein Suggestions for Day 13 Lunch and Dinner

Same as Day 11.

Vegetable Suggestions for Day 13 Lunch and Dinner

Same as Day 11.

Fruit Suggestions for Day 13

Same as Day 11.

SUPPLEMENTS

Take:

○ Vitamin C, 1000 mg per day in the morning.

○ Co Q 10, 120 mg per day in the morning **and at 4 P.M.**

○ Omega-3 DHA and EPA, 300 mg per day in the morning and at 4 P.M.

○ Vitamin B complex, 100 mg per day in the morning.

○ L-carnitine, 500 mg in the morning and 500 mg at 4 P.M.

EXERCISE

Same as Day 11.

DAILY JOURNAL

Calendar Day_____

Day of Cycle_____

(Day 1 = Start of Period)

DIET

BREAKFAST	Time	Amount	Food Brand

LUNCH	Time	Amount	Food Brand

DINNER	Time	Amount	Food Brand

SNACKS	Time	Amount	Food Brand

LIQUIDS	Type	Amount

EXERCISE

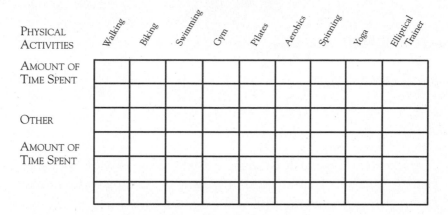

PHYSICAL ACTIVITIES	Walking	Biking	Swimming	Gym	Pilates	Aerobics	Spinning	Yoga	Elliptical Trainer
AMOUNT OF TIME SPENT									
OTHER									
AMOUNT OF TIME SPENT									

LIFESTYLE

WORK/SCHOOL	Gratifying	Satisfying	Rewarding	Exciting	Stressful	Boring	Terrible	N/A
RELATIONSHIPS	Gratifying	Satisfying	Rewarding	Exciting	Stressful	Boring	Terrible	N/A
MOOD	Good		Indifferent		Bad		Other	
SLEEP (NUMBER OF HOURS)	Continuous		Interrupted					
STRESS LEVEL (RATE 1–5)								
OVERALL RATING OF THE DAY								
(RATE 1–5)								

1=EXCELLENT

5=POOR

DAY 14

NATURAL HORMONES

Same as Day 11.

DIET

○ Drink water. **Have at least eight glasses today—unless you just ovulated, in which case you should start decreasing water intake to six glasses maximum until you get your period.**

○ Drink at least one cup of green tea today.

Breakfast

Same as Day 11.

Snacks

○ Same as Day 11.

○ **1 hard-boiled egg.**

Lunch and Dinner

○ Before lunch and dinner, drink an eight-ounce glass of water, and then wait ten minutes before eating.

○ At least once today, include Erika's Favorite Anytime Salad (page 142).

○ No alcoholic beverages.

○ Reduce the number of sodas you drink (diet or regular) by half again.

○ Reduce the amount of bread and potatoes you eat by half.

Protein Suggestions for Day 14 Lunch and Dinner

Same as Day 11.

Vegetable Suggestions for Day 14 Lunch and Dinner

Same as Day 11.

Fruit Suggestions for Day 14

Same as Day 11.

SUPPLEMENTS

Take:

- Vitamin C, 1000 mg per day in the morning.
- Co Q 10, 120 mg per day in the morning and at 4 P.M.
- Omega-3 DHA and EPA, 300 mg per day in the morning and at 4 P.M.
- Vitamin B complex, 100 mg per day in the morning.
- L-carnitine, 500 mg in the morning and 500 mg at 4 P.M.
- **Calcium 1000 mg, magnesium 400 mg, and zinc 25 mg, all in one pill, in the evening before going to sleep.**

EXERCISE

Same as Day 11.

DAILY JOURNAL

Calendar Day_____

Day of Cycle_____

(Day 1 = Start of Period)

DIET

BREAKFAST	Time	Amount	Food Brand
LUNCH	Time	Amount	Food Brand
DINNER	Time	Amount	Food Brand
SNACKS	Time	Amount	Food Brand
LIQUIDS	Type	Amount	

EXERCISE

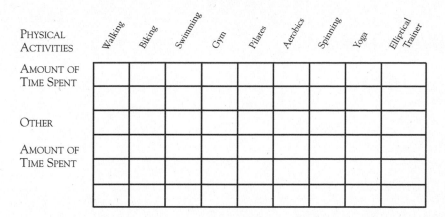

Physical Activities	Walking	Biking	Swimming	Gym	Pilates	Aerobics	Spinning	Yoga	Elliptical Trainer
Amount of Time Spent									
Other									
Amount of Time Spent									

LIFESTYLE

Work/School	Gratifying	Satisfying	Rewarding	Exciting	Stressful	Boring	Terrible	N/A
Relationships	Gratifying	Satisfying	Rewarding	Exciting	Stressful	Boring	Terrible	N/A
Mood	Good		Indifferent		Bad		Other	
Sleep (Number of Hours)	Continuous		Interrupted					
Stress Level (Rate 1–5)								
Overall Rating of the Day								
(Rate 1–5)								

1=Excellent

5=Poor

DAY 15

NATURAL HORMONES

Same as Day 11.

DIET

○ Drink water. Have at least eight glasses today.

○ Drink at least one cup of green tea.

Breakfast

Same as Day 11.

Snacks

Include a snack two or three hours after both breakfast and lunch. For each snack, choose one:

○ ½ scoop Metagenics UltraClear in 1 glass of orange juice or water.

○ Protein bar.

○ Designer Whey Protein drink.

○ 1 hard-boiled egg.

○ **1 apple, plum, or pear with 2 slices rye melba toast and tea.**

Lunch and Dinner

- Before lunch and dinner, drink an eight-ounce glass of water, and then wait ten minutes before eating.

- At least once today, include Erika's Favorite Anytime Salad (page 142).

- No alcoholic beverages.

- Keep reducing the number of sodas you drink (diet or regular) by half.

- Keep reducing the amount of bread and potatoes you consume.

Protein Suggestions for Day 15 Lunch and Dinner

Same as Day 11.

Vegetable Suggestions for Day 15 Lunch and Dinner

Same as Day 11.

Fruit Suggestions for Day 15.

Same as Day 11.

SUPPLEMENTS

Take:

- Vitamin C, 1000 mg per day in the morning.
- Co Q 10, 120 mg per day in the morning and at 4 P.M.

○ Omega-3 DHA and EPA, 300 mg per day in the morning and at
  4 P.M.

○ Vitamin B complex, 100 mg per day in the morning.

○ L-carnitine, 500 mg in the morning and 500 mg at 4 P.M.

○ Calcium 1000 mg, magnesium 400 mg, and zinc 25 mg, all in one
  pill, in the evening before going to sleep.

EXERCISE

Same as Day 11.

DAILY JOURNAL

Calendar Day_____

Day of Cycle_____

(Day 1 = Start of Period)

DIET

BREAKFAST	Time	Amount	Food Brand
LUNCH	Time	Amount	Food Brand
DINNER	Time	Amount	Food Brand
SNACKS	Time	Amount	Food Brand
LIQUIDS	Type	Amount	

EXERCISE

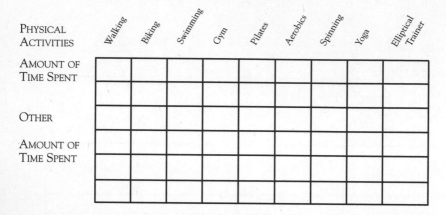

PHYSICAL ACTIVITIES	Walking	Biking	Swimming	Gym	Pilates	Aerobics	Spinning	Yoga	Elliptical Trainer
AMOUNT OF TIME SPENT									
OTHER									
AMOUNT OF TIME SPENT									

LIFESTYLE

WORK/SCHOOL	Gratifying	Satisfying	Rewarding	Exciting	Stressful	Boring	Terrible	N/A
RELATIONSHIPS	Gratifying	Satisfying	Rewarding	Exciting	Stressful	Boring	Terrible	N/A
MOOD	Good		Indifferent		Bad		Other	
SLEEP (NUMBER OF HOURS)	Continuous		Interrupted					
STRESS LEVEL (RATE 1–5)								
OVERALL RATING OF THE DAY (RATE 1–5)								

1=EXCELLENT

5=POOR

13

◯

Keep Up the Good Work:
Days 16–20

Congratulations—you're now past the halfway mark! It hasn't been that difficult, has it? I know, because I follow the plan myself. I also see hundreds of patients every month who are happily working on following the plan, and they invariably tell me that it's magical. Whenever I slip up (I fall into the human being category, too—more than you know), I go back to Week 1 and start again. It doesn't take me thirty days to get up to speed again; usually I feel back to normal within seven to ten days.

Now that you've gotten into the swing of things, you can kick it up a notch. If you want to increase your exercise beyond what I have listed here, feel free (as long as you check out any intended exercise program with your physician first). The recommendations I list here are suggestions for minimum amounts. The more you do (within reason), the better you'll feel. If you're a beginner, you'll want to stay with the pace in these pages. If you exercise regularly, you may want to use these suggestions as a foundation and add more activity. Choose the path that works best for you. This is not a race, and it's not a comparison with how anyone else is doing. This is something you're doing for yourself and for your own body. If your body tells you to take it slowly, then take it slowly. If you feel you can do more, then go ahead. Just don't be impatient. Enjoy the results, and don't get ahead of yourself.

DAY 16

NATURAL HORMONES

Estradiol 0.6 mg and micronized progesterone 200 mg per day in divided doses, preferably in cream form.

Take this opportunity to assess how you're doing on the hormones. If you feel you need to adjust the dosage, discuss this with your doctor. And remember, do not take the hormones while you have your period.

DIET

○ Drink water. Have at least eight glasses today.

○ Drink at least one cup of green tea today.

Breakfast

Have one slice of multigrain toast and a six-ounce glass of orange or grapefruit juice. In addition, choose from:

○ Oz Garcia's Favorite Smoothie (page 140).

○ Three-Egg Omelet (page 164).

○ Three-Egg Vegetable Omelet (follow the recipe on page 164, but add 1 cup of your favorite vegetables: steamed spinach, broccoli, mushrooms, peppers, or onions).

○ 1 cup oatmeal in ½ cup skimmed milk, rice milk, or soy milk.

○ **Poach 2 eggs in water and pour over a plate of steamed spinach.**

○ **1 cup cottage cheese with a few slices of cantaloupe, apples, and/or berries.**

Snacks

Include a snack two or three hours after both breakfast and lunch. For each snack, choose one:

- ½ scoop Metagenics UltraClear in 1 glass of orange juice or water.
- Protein bar.
- Designer Whey Protein drink.
- 1 hard-boiled egg.
- 1 apple, plum, or pear with 2 slices rye melba toast and tea.
- **Cottage cheese with fruit (for instance 1 cup berries, half an apple, or half a banana).**
- **1 cup yogurt with berries and granola.**

Lunch and Dinner

- Before lunch and dinner, drink an eight-ounce glass of water, and then wait ten minutes before eating.
- At least once today, include Erika's Favorite Anytime Salad (page 142).
- No alcoholic beverages.
- **Eliminate all soda.**
- **No fast foods.**

Protein Suggestions for Day 16 Lunch and Dinner

- ¼ pound turkey breast.
- 1 can tuna fish packed in water.
- 1 chicken breast.

- 1 cup tofu.

- 8 ounces salmon, baked, grilled, or poached.

- 8–10 pieces of sushi.

- **6–8-ounce lean steak, rib or sirloin cut.**

Vegetable Suggestion for Day 16 Lunch and Dinner

Have any vegetable listed under "Fiber" in chapter 5. Here are some ways to spice them up:

- 1 cup diced white or red cabbage with 3 tablespoons white vinegar and 1 tablespoon olive oil, salted to taste.

- 1 cup steamed broccoli with 1 tablespoon olive oil and a few drops of lemon, salted to taste.

- 1 cup steamed spinach with 1 tablespoon olive oil and a little salt and lemon.

- 1 cup steamed brussels sprouts with 1 tablespoon olive oil, 1 garlic clove, salt, and pepper.

- ½ head steamed cabbage with 1 tablespoon olive oil, 1 crushed garlic clove, salt, and pepper.

- ½ head Boston or 2 cups romaine, red leaf, arugula, or dandelion lettuce, 1 tomato, 1 slice onion (chopped), 1 tablespoon olive oil, 1 tablespoon balsamic vinegar, salt and pepper to taste.

- 1 cup steamed beets with salt and pepper and a touch of red wine vinegar.

- 1 cup green beans steamed with 1 cup tomato sauce, ¼ teaspoon oregano, ¼ teaspoon chopped fresh dill, 1 tablespoon olive oil, 1 crushed small garlic clove, and ½ onion (diced).

- **1 cup beets, parboiled, salted, and with a drop of red wine vinegar and 1 teaspoon olive oil.**

Fruit Suggestions for Day 16

Do not have more than two fruits a day, and do not eat fruit by itself before noon. Choose from:

- 1 apple.
- 1 apricot.
- 1 banana.
- ½ medium cantaloupe.
- 2 medium slices honeydew melon.
- 2 cups cherries.
- 1 medium orange.
- 2 small tangerines.
- 1 mango.
- 1 peach.
- 1 medium pear.
- **2 mandarin oranges.**
- **½ cup grapes.**

SUPPLEMENTS

Take:

- Vitamin C, 1000 mg per day in the morning.
- Co Q 10, 120 mg per day in the morning and at 4 P.M.
- Omega-3 DHA and EPA, 300 mg per day in the morning and at 4 P.M.
- Vitamin B complex, 100 mg per day in the morning.
- L-carnitine, 500 mg in the morning and 500 mg at 4 P.M.

○ Calcium 1000 mg, magnesium 400 mg, and zinc 25 mg, all in one pill, in the evening before going to sleep.

EXERCISE

○ In the morning: start your day with ten minutes of stretching.

○ **Walk briskly for thirty to forty-five minutes today.**

○ **Do fifteen crunches:** Lie with your back on the floor, your legs bent, and your feet flat on the floor. Clasp your hands behind your head. Do not pull on your neck. Keep your back as flat on the floor as possible. Curl your upper body forward and hold for ten seconds. Lift your shoulder blades off the floor three inches. As you come up, look up toward the highest point you have risen to. Don't keep your eyes fixed on one point. Don't forget to breathe.

○ **Do fifteen side bends:** Begin by standing up straight, knees slightly bent. Drop your head to the left. Once you feel a stretch in your neck, gently slide your left hand down your leg toward the floor. Breathe. You should feel the stretch in your right side. Do not pull on your neck. Hold this position for ten seconds. Slowly roll back up. Repeat on the right side.

○ **Do ten leg raises:** Lie on your back, with your back as flat on the floor as possible. (Use a yoga mat or towel.) Bend your left leg and keep your left foot flat on the floor. Keep your right leg straight, foot flexed, knee slightly bent. Pull in your stomach muscles (think of your belly button reaching your back through your belly) and slowly raise your right leg to a forty-five degree angle. Breathe out and lower your leg to a count of ten. Repeat on the other leg.

○ In the middle of the day: **Add ten Kegel exercises to the previous routine—you are now doing Kegels four times a day.** (Tighten your vagina, hold it closed for a count of ten, and breathe.)

○ Sit straight in your chair and suck in your abdominal muscles to the count of twenty. Breathe. **Repeat every four hours.**

○ **While sitting, tighten your butt, count to ten, breathe, release. Repeat ten times, at least three times a day.**

○ Include some aerobic exercises in your routine. Refer to chapter 6 to determine which ones are appropriate for your age group. If you haven't exercised in a while, start slowly and gently. Many gyms now offer nonimpact aerobic classes, which are easier on older joints.

○ **Get a three-pound weight. Hold it in your right hand, palm facing up. Straighten your arm out to the side (keep elbows soft), then lift it five times above your head. Repeat using the other arm (you can use a liter bottle of water instead of the weight).**

○ After dinner: If you ate out, walk for fifteen minutes before getting into your car. If that's not possible, go home and walk around your house for fifteen minutes. If you have stairs, walk up and down them for fifteen minutes.

○ If you ate at home, do not go sit on the couch as soon as you finish eating. Walk up and down two flights of stairs or around the room twenty times.

○ Do not do serious aerobic or stressful exercises after dinner; you may release adrenaline and endorphins which will keep you awake.

○ **Take ten minutes today for quiet time—meditation, personal yoga, or whatever works for you. Find a quiet place, even if it's in the bathroom. Sit down without slouching and close your eyes. Visualize something you love—a beach, a forest, calming music, whatever. Then think of health permeating every cell of your body. Feel the negative energy leaving through your fingers, nose, and toes and the good energy overtaking your whole body. Start with three cleansing breaths and end with three cleansing breaths. Use this in your life whenever you feel overwhelmed, scared, or angry.**

DAILY JOURNAL

Calendar Day_____

Day of Cycle_____

(Day 1 = Start of Period)

DIET

BREAKFAST	Time	Amount	Food Brand
LUNCH	Time	Amount	Food Brand
DINNER	Time	Amount	Food Brand
SNACKS	Time	Amount	Food Brand
LIQUIDS	Type	Amount	

EXERCISE

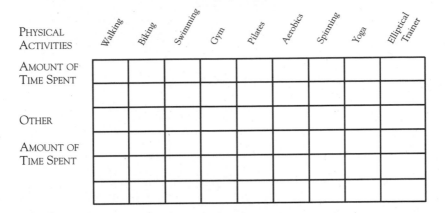

PHYSICAL ACTIVITIES	Walking	Biking	Swimming	Gym	Pilates	Aerobics	Spinning	Yoga	Elliptical Trainer
AMOUNT OF TIME SPENT									
OTHER									
AMOUNT OF TIME SPENT									

LIFESTYLE

WORK/SCHOOL	Gratifying	Satisfying	Rewarding	Exciting	Stressful	Boring	Terrible	N/A
RELATIONSHIPS	Gratifying	Satisfying	Rewarding	Exciting	Stressful	Boring	Terrible	N/A
MOOD	Good		Indifferent		Bad		Other	
SLEEP (NUMBER OF HOURS)	Continuous		Interrupted					
STRESS LEVEL (RATE 1–5)								
OVERALL RATING OF THE DAY								
(RATE 1–5)								

1=EXCELLENT

5=POOR

DAY 17

NATURAL HORMONES

Same as Day 16.

DIET

○ Drink water. Have at least eight glasses today.
○ Drink at least one cup of green tea today.

Breakfast

Same as Day 16.

Snacks

Same as Day 16.

Lunch and Dinner

Same as Day 16.

Protein Suggestions for Day 17 Lunch and Dinner

Same as Day 16.

Vegetable Suggestions for Day 17 Lunch and Dinner

Same as Day 16.

Fruit Suggestions for Day 17

Same as Day 16.

SUPPLEMENTS

Same as Day 16.

EXERCISE

Same as Day 16.

DAILY JOURNAL

Calendar Day_____

Day of Cycle_____

(Day 1 = Start of Period)

DIET

BREAKFAST	Time	Amount	Food Brand

LUNCH	Time	Amount	Food Brand

DINNER	Time	Amount	Food Brand

SNACKS	Time	Amount	Food Brand

LIQUIDS	Type	Amount	

EXERCISE

PHYSICAL ACTIVITIES	Walking	Biking	Swimming	Gym	Pilates	Aerobics	Spinning	Yoga	Elliptical Trainer
AMOUNT OF TIME SPENT									
OTHER									
AMOUNT OF TIME SPENT									

LIFESTYLE

WORK/SCHOOL	Gratifying	Satisfying	Rewarding	Exciting	Stressful	Boring	Terrible	N/A
RELATIONSHIPS	Gratifying	Satisfying	Rewarding	Exciting	Stressful	Boring	Terrible	N/A
MOOD	Good		Indifferent		Bad		Other	
SLEEP (NUMBER OF HOURS)	Continuous		Interrupted					
STRESS LEVEL (RATE 1–5)								

OVERALL RATING OF THE DAY								
(RATE 1–5)								

1=EXCELLENT

5=POOR

DAY 18

NATURAL HORMONES

Same as Day 16.

DIET

○ Drink water. Have at least eight glasses today.
○ Drink at least one cup of green tea today.

Breakfast

Same as Day 16.

Snacks

Same as Day 16.

Lunch and Dinner

Same as Day 16.

Protein Suggestions for Day 18 Lunch and Dinner

Same as Day 16.

Vegetable Suggestions for Day 18 Lunch and Dinner

Same as Day 16.

Fruit Suggestions for Day 18

Same as Day 16.

SUPPLEMENTS

Same as Day 16.

EXERCISE

Same as Day 16.

DAILY JOURNAL

Calendar Day_____

Day of Cycle_____

(Day 1 = Start of Period)

DIET

BREAKFAST	Time	Amount	Food Brand
LUNCH	Time	Amount	Food Brand
DINNER	Time	Amount	Food Brand
SNACKS	Time	Amount	Food Brand
LIQUIDS	Type	Amount	

EXERCISE

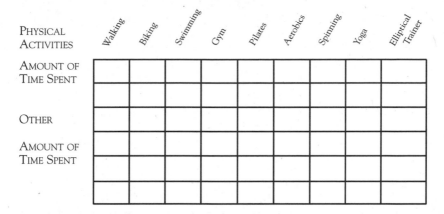

Physical Activities	Walking	Biking	Swimming	Gym	Pilates	Aerobics	Spinning	Yoga	Elliptical Trainer
Amount of Time Spent									
Other									
Amount of Time Spent									

LIFESTYLE

Work/School	Gratifying	Satisfying	Rewarding	Exciting	Stressful	Boring	Terrible	N/A
Relationships	Gratifying	Satisfying	Rewarding	Exciting	Stressful	Boring	Terrible	N/A
Mood	Good		Indifferent		Bad		Other	
Sleep (Number of Hours)	Continuous		Interrupted					
Stress Level (Rate 1–5)								

Overall Rating of the Day							
(Rate 1–5)							

1=Excellent

5=Poor

DAY 19

NATURAL HORMONES

Same as Day 16.

DIET

○ Drink six to eight glasses of water.

○ **Increase your tea intake; it is a diuretic, so you should now drink a cup of green or other tea three times a day. Have the last cup before 6 P.M.**

Breakfast

Same as Day 16.

Snacks

Same as Day 16.

Lunch and Dinner

○ Same as Day 16.

○ **Reduce the number of fried or highly spiced foods you eat per week.**

Protein Suggestions for Day 19 Lunch and Dinner

Same as Day 16.

Vegetable Suggestions for Day 19 Lunch and Dinner

Same as Day 16.

Fruit Suggestions for Day 19

Same as Day 16.

SUPPLEMENTS

Same as Day 16.

EXERCISE

Same as Day 16.

DAILY JOURNAL

Calendar Day_____

Day of Cycle_____

(Day 1 = Start of Period)

DIET

BREAKFAST	Time	Amount	Food Brand

LUNCH	Time	Amount	Food Brand

DINNER	Time	Amount	Food Brand

SNACKS	Time	Amount	Food Brand

LIQUIDS	Type	Amount	

EXERCISE

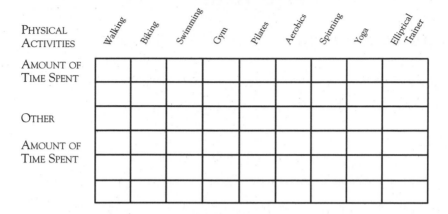

Physical Activities	Walking	Biking	Swimming	Gym	Pilates	Aerobics	Spinning	Yoga	Elliptical Trainer
Amount of Time Spent									
Other									
Amount of Time Spent									

LIFESTYLE

Work/School	Gratifying	Satisfying	Rewarding	Exciting	Stressful	Boring	Terrible	N/A
Relationships	Gratifying	Satisfying	Rewarding	Exciting	Stressful	Boring	Terrible	N/A
Mood	Good		Indifferent		Bad		Other	
Sleep (Number of Hours)	Continuous		Interrupted					
Stress Level (Rate 1–5)								
Overall Rating of the Day								
(Rate 1–5)								

1=Excellent

5=Poor

DAY 20

NATURAL HORMONES

Same as Day 16.

DIET

○ Drink six to eight glasses of water.

○ Drink at least three cups of green or other tea today.

Breakfast

Same as Day 16.

Snacks

○ Same as Day 16.

○ **10 roasted, unsalted, almonds along with 10 pieces of dried apricots, plums, or pears.**

Lunch and Dinner

Same as Day 16.

Protein Suggestions for Day 20 Lunch and Dinner

Same as Day 16.

Vegetable Suggestions for Day 20 Lunch and Dinner

Same as Day 16.

Fruit Suggestions for Day 20

Same as Day 16.

SUPPLEMENTS

Same as Day 16.

EXERCISE

○ Same as Day 16.

   Also, add one of the following:

○ **A yoga class, spinning class, or Pilates class.**

○ **A weekly massage.**

○ **A weekly relaxation bath or sauna.**

DAILY JOURNAL

Calendar Day_____

Day of Cycle_____

(Day 1 = Start of Period)

DIET

BREAKFAST	Time	Amount	Food Brand
LUNCH	Time	Amount	Food Brand
DINNER	Time	Amount	Food Brand
SNACKS	Time	Amount	Food Brand
LIQUIDS	Type	Amount	

EXERCISE

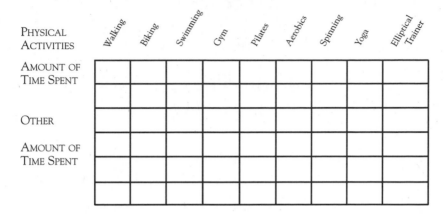

Physical Activities	Walking	Biking	Swimming	Gym	Pilates	Aerobics	Spinning	Yoga	Elliptical Trainer
Amount of Time Spent									
Other									
Amount of Time Spent									

LIFESTYLE

Work/School	Gratifying	Satisfying	Rewarding	Exciting	Stressful	Boring	Terrible	N/A
Relationships	Gratifying	Satisfying	Rewarding	Exciting	Stressful	Boring	Terrible	N/A
Mood	Good		Indifferent		Bad		Other	
Sleep (Number of Hours)	Continuous		Interrupted					
Stress Level (Rate 1–5)								
Overall Rating of the Day								
(Rate 1–5)								

1=Excellent

5=Poor

14

◯

Almost There:
Days 21–25

Now that you're three weeks into the program and your habits are beginning to change, there are a few things I should mention that I haven't discussed before. One has to do with diet and portion size. I've given you guidelines where protein, fruits, and vegetables are concerned. But how do you know the true amounts of the foods you're eating?

You don't always know. Obviously, when you cook at home, you can weigh and measure your food. But what about when you eat out? First, remember that size matters. You want your cells to be able to make good energy, maintain your hormones in balance, keep your blood sugar levels even, and keep insulin at bay. The best way to accomplish all these things is to eat reasonable portions at frequent intervals during the day. This might mean making your lunch or dinner meals smaller and adding more to your snacks. Try it and see how it makes you feel. Try eating your largest meal at lunchtime (if this fits in with your lifestyle). Even if you can't do it every day, you may be able to manage several times a week. Now is the time to try new things just to see what effect they have on how you feel overall.

DAY 21

NATURAL HORMONES

Estradiol 0.6 mg and micronized progesterone 200 mg per day in divided doses, preferably in cream form.

DIET

○ Drink water. Have at least six to eight glasses today.

○ Drink at least three cups of green or other tea today.

Breakfast

Have one slice of multigrain toast and a six-ounce glass of orange or grapefruit juice. In addition, choose from:

○ Oz Garcia's Favorite Smoothie (page 140).

○ Three-Egg Omelet (page 164).

○ Three-Egg Vegetable Omelet (follow the recipe on page 164, but add 1 cup of your favorite vegetables: steamed spinach, broccoli, mushrooms, peppers, or onions).

○ 1 cup oatmeal in ½ cup skimmed milk, rice milk, or soy milk.

○ Poach 2 eggs in water and pour over a plate of steamed spinach.

○ **1 cup cottage cheese with a few slices of cantaloupe, apples, and/or berries, along with some granola, Total, or other high-fiber, high-protein, low-carbohydrate cereal.**

○ **Yogurt, fruit, and granola.**

Snacks

Include a snack two or three hours after both breakfast and lunch. For each snack, choose one:

- ½ scoop Metagenics UltraClear in 1 glass of orange juice or water.

- Protein bar.

- Designer Whey Protein drink.

- **2 hard-boiled eggs.**

- 1 apple, plum, or pear with 2 slices rye melba toast and tea.

- Low-fat cottage cheese with fruit (for instance 1 cup of berries, half an apple, or half a banana).

- 1 cup low-fat yogurt with berries and granola.

- 10 roasted, unsalted almonds, along with 10 pieces of dried apricots, plums, or pears.

- **3 cubes feta, cheddar, or other hard cheese and 3 high-fiber, low-carbohydrate, low-fat crackers.**

Lunch and Dinner

- Before lunch and dinner, drink an eight-ounce glass of water, and then wait ten minutes before eating.

- At least once today, include Erika's Favorite Anytime Salad (page 142).

- No alcoholic beverages.

- Eliminate all soda.

- No fast foods.

- Reduce the number of fried or highly spiced foods you eat per week.

- **Have no more than one pasta meal or serving of potatoes for the whole week.**

Protein Suggestions for Day 21 Lunch and Dinner

- ¼ pound turkey breast.

- 1 can tuna fish packed in water.

- 1 chicken breast.

- 1 cup tofu.

- 8 ounces salmon, baked, grilled, or poached.

- 8–10 pieces of sushi.

- 6- to 8-ounce lean steak—rib or sirloin cut.

Vegetable Suggestions for Day 21 Lunch and Dinner

Have any vegetable listed under "Fiber" in chapter 5. Here are some ways to spice them up:

- 1 cup diced white or red cabbage with 3 tablespoons white vinegar and 1 tablespoon olive oil, salted to taste.

- 1 cup steamed broccoli with 1 tablespoon olive oil and a few drops of lemon, salted to taste.

- 1 cup steamed spinach with 1 tablespoon olive oil and a little salt and lemon.

- 1 cup steamed brussels sprouts with 1 tablespoon olive oil, 1 crushed garlic clove, salt, and pepper.

❑ ½ head steamed cabbage with 1 tablespoon olive oil, 1 crushed garlic clove, salt, and pepper.

❑ ½ head Boston or 2 cups romaine, red leaf, arugula, or dandelion lettuce, 1 tomato, 1 slice onion (chopped), 1 tablespoon olive oil, 1 tablespoon balsamic vinegar, salt and pepper to taste.

❑ 1 cup steamed beets with salt and pepper and a touch of red wine vinegar.

❑ 1 cup green beans steamed with 1 cup tomato sauce, ¼ teaspoon oregano, ¼ teaspoon chopped fresh dill, 1 tablespoon olive oil, 1 crushed small garlic clove, and ½ onion (diced).

❑ 1 cup beets, parboiled, salted, and with a drop of red wine vinegar.

❑ **1 cup boiled, mashed yams, flavored with nutmeg and 1 teaspoon brown sugar and baked in a 325-degree oven for 15 minutes.**

Fruit Suggestions for Day 21

Do not have more than two fruits a day, and do not eat fruit by itself before noon. Choose from:

❑ 1 apple.

❑ 1 apricot.

❑ 1 banana.

❑ ½ medium cantaloupe.

❑ 2 medium slices honeydew melon.

❑ 2 cups cherries.

❑ 1 medium orange.

❑ 2 small tangerines.

❑ 1 mango.

- 1 peach.
- 1 medium pear.
- 2 mandarin oranges.
- ½ cup grapes.
- **1 passion fruit.**

SUPPLEMENTS

Take:

- Vitamin C, 1000 mg today in the morning.
- Co Q 10, 120 mg today in the morning and at 4 P.M.
- Omega-3 DHA and EPA, 300 mg today in the morning and at 4 P.M.
- Vitamin B complex, 100 mg today in the morning.
- L-carnitine, 500 mg in the morning and 500 mg at 4 P.M.
- Calcium 1000 mg, magnesium 400 mg, and zinc 25 mg, all in one pill, in the evening before going to sleep.

EXERCISE

- In the morning: Start your day with ten minutes of stretching.
- Walk for thirty to forty-five minutes today; **increase your pace to a fifteen- to twenty-minute mile.**

○ Do twenty crunches: Lie with your back on the floor, your legs bent, and your feet flat on the floor. Clasp your hands behind your head. Keep your back as flat to the floor as possible. Curl your upper body forward and hold for five seconds. Don't forget to breathe.

○ Do twenty side bends: Begin by standing up straight. Drop your head to the left. Once you feel a stretch in your neck, gently slide your left hand down your leg toward the floor. Breathe. You should feel the stretch in your right side. Hold this position for five seconds. Slowly roll back up. Repeat on the other side.

○ Do eight to twelve biceps curls: Stand with a pair of three-pound dumbbells in your hands, palms facing front and feet shoulder width apart. Keeping your elbows stable, raise the dumbbells toward your shoulders and bring them back down slowly. You can also do this exercise while seated.

○ After dinner: If you ate out, walk for fifteen minutes before getting into your car. If that's not possible, go home and walk around your house for fifteen minutes. If you have stairs, walk up and down them for fifteen minutes.

○ If you ate at home, do not go sit on the couch as soon as you finish eating. Walk up and down two flights of stairs or around the room twenty times.

○ Do not do serious aerobic or stressful exercises after dinner; you may release adrenaline and endorphins, which will keep you awake.

○ Take ten minutes today for quiet time—meditation, personal yoga, or whatever works for you. Find a quiet place, even if it's in the bathroom. Sit down without slouching and close your eyes. Visualize something you love—a beach, a forest, calming music, whatever. Then think of health permeating every cell of your body. Feel the negative energy leaving through your fingers, nose, and toes and the good energy overtaking your whole body.

Start with three cleansing breaths and end with three cleansing breaths. Use this in your life whenever you feel overwhelmed, scared, or angry.

○ Include one of the following in your routine each week: a yoga, spinning, or Pilates class; a massage; or a relaxation bath or sauna.

DAILY JOURNAL

Calendar Day_____

Day of Cycle_____

(Day 1 = Start of Period)

DIET

BREAKFAST	Time	Amount	Food Brand
LUNCH	Time	Amount	Food Brand
DINNER	Time	Amount	Food Brand
SNACKS	Time	Amount	Food Brand
LIQUIDS	Type	Amount	

EXERCISE

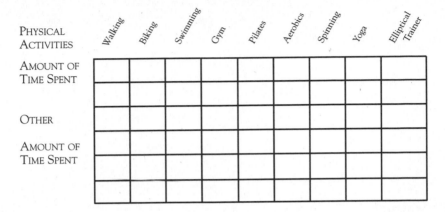

PHYSICAL ACTIVITIES	Walking	Biking	Swimming	Gym	Pilates	Aerobics	Spinning	Yoga	Elliptical Trainer
AMOUNT OF TIME SPENT									
OTHER									
AMOUNT OF TIME SPENT									

LIFESTYLE

WORK/SCHOOL	Gratifying	Satisfying	Rewarding	Exciting	Stressful	Boring	Terrible	N/A
RELATIONSHIPS	Gratifying	Satisfying	Rewarding	Exciting	Stressful	Boring	Terrible	N/A
MOOD	Good		Indifferent		Bad		Other	
SLEEP (NUMBER OF HOURS)	Continuous		Interrupted					
STRESS LEVEL (RATE 1–5)								
OVERALL RATING OF THE DAY								
(RATE 1–5)								

1=EXCELLENT

5=POOR

DAY 22

NATURAL HORMONES

Same as Day 21.

DIET

○ Drink water. Have at least six to eight glasses today.
○ Drink at least three cups of green or other tea today.

Breakfast

Same as Day 21.

Snacks

Same as Day 21.

Lunch and Dinner

Same as Day 21.

Protein Suggestions for Day 22 Lunch and Dinner

Same as Day 21.

Vegetable Suggestions for Day 22 Lunch and Dinner

Same as Day 21.

Fruit Suggestions for Day 22

Same as Day 21.

SUPPLEMENTS

Same as Day 21.

EXERCISE

Same as Day 21.

DAILY JOURNAL

Calendar Day_____

Day of Cycle_____

(Day 1 = Start of Period)

DIET

BREAKFAST	Time	Amount	Food Brand
LUNCH	Time	Amount	Food Brand
DINNER	Time	Amount	Food Brand
SNACKS	Time	Amount	Food Brand
LIQUIDS	Type	Amount	

EXERCISE

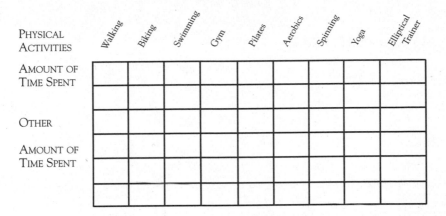

Physical Activities	Walking	Biking	Swimming	Gym	Pilates	Aerobics	Spinning	Yoga	Elliptical Trainer
Amount of Time Spent									
Other									
Amount of Time Spent									

LIFESTYLE

Work/School	Gratifying	Satisfying	Rewarding	Exciting	Stressful	Boring	Terrible	N/A
Relationships	Gratifying	Satisfying	Rewarding	Exciting	Stressful	Boring	Terrible	N/A
Mood	Good		Indifferent		Bad		Other	
Sleep (Number of Hours)	Continuous		Interrupted					
Stress Level (Rate 1–5)								
Overall Rating of the Day								
(Rate 1–5)								

1=Excellent

5=Poor

DAY 23

NATURAL HORMONES

Same as Day 21.

DIET

○ Drink water. Have at least six to eight glasses today.
○ Drink at least three cups of green or other tea today.

Breakfast

Same as Day 21.

Snacks

Same as Day 21.

Lunch and Dinner

Same as Day 21.

Protein Suggestions for Day 23 Lunch and Dinner

Same as Day 21.

Vegetable Suggestions for Day 23 Lunch and Dinner

Same as Day 21.

Fruit Suggestions for Day 23

Same as Day 21.

SUPPLEMENTS

Same as Day 21.

EXERCISE

Same as Day 21.

DAILY JOURNAL

Calendar Day_____

Day of Cycle_____

(Day 1 = Start of Period)

DIET

BREAKFAST	Time	Amount	Food Brand
LUNCH	Time	Amount	Food Brand
DINNER	Time	Amount	Food Brand
SNACKS	Time	Amount	Food Brand
LIQUIDS	Type	Amount	

EXERCISE

PHYSICAL ACTIVITIES	Walking	Biking	Swimming	Gym	Pilates	Aerobics	Spinning	Yoga	Elliptical Trainer
AMOUNT OF TIME SPENT									
OTHER									
AMOUNT OF TIME SPENT									

LIFESTYLE

WORK/SCHOOL	Gratifying	Satisfying	Rewarding	Exciting	Stressful	Boring	Terrible	N/A
RELATIONSHIPS	Gratifying	Satisfying	Rewarding	Exciting	Stressful	Boring	Terrible	N/A
MOOD	Good		Indifferent		Bad		Other	
SLEEP (NUMBER OF HOURS)	Continuous		Interrupted					
STRESS LEVEL (RATE 1–5)								
OVERALL RATING OF THE DAY								
(RATE 1–5)								

1=EXCELLENT

5=POOR

DAY 24

NATURAL HORMONES

Same as Day 21.

DIET

- Drink water. Have at least six to eight glasses today.
- Drink at least three cups of green or other tea today.

Breakfast

Same as Day 21.

Snacks

Same as Day 21.

Lunch and Dinner

Same as Day 21.

Protein Suggestions for Day 24 Lunch and Dinner

Same as Day 21.

Vegetable Suggestions for Day 24 Lunch and Dinner

Same as Day 21.

Fruit Suggestions for Day 24

Same as Day 21.

SUPPLEMENTS

Same as Day 21.

EXERCISE

Same as Day 21.

DAILY JOURNAL

Calendar Day_____

Day of Cycle_____

(Day 1 = Start of Period)

DIET

BREAKFAST	Time	Amount	Food Brand
LUNCH	Time	Amount	Food Brand
DINNER	Time	Amount	Food Brand
SNACKS	Time	Amount	Food Brand
LIQUIDS	Type	Amount	

EXERCISE

Physical Activities	Walking	Biking	Swimming	Gym	Pilates	Aerobics	Spinning	Yoga	Elliptical Trainer
Amount of Time Spent									
Other									
Amount of Time Spent									

LIFESTYLE

Work/School	Gratifying	Satisfying	Rewarding	Exciting	Stressful	Boring	Terrible	N/A
Relationships	Gratifying	Satisfying	Rewarding	Exciting	Stressful	Boring	Terrible	N/A
Mood	Good		Indifferent		Bad		Other	
Sleep (Number of Hours)	Continuous		Interrupted					
Stress Level (Rate 1–5)								
Overall Rating of the Day								
(Rate 1–5)								

1=Excellent

5=Poor

DAY 25

NATURAL HORMONES

Same as Day 21.

DIET

○ Drink water. Have at least six to eight glasses today.
○ Drink at least three cups of green or other tea today.

Breakfast

Same as Day 21.

Snacks

Same as Day 21.

Lunch and Dinner

Same as Day 21.

Protein Suggestions for Day 25 Lunch and Dinner

Same as Day 21.

Vegetable Suggestions for Day 25 Lunch and Dinner

Same as Day 21.

Fruit Suggestions for Day 25

Same as Day 21.

SUPPLEMENTS

Same as Day 21.

EXERCISE

Same as Day 21.

DAILY JOURNAL

Calendar Day_____

Day of Cycle_____

(Day 1 = Start of Period)

DIET

BREAKFAST	Time	Amount	Food Brand
LUNCH	Time	Amount	Food Brand
DINNER	Time	Amount	Food Brand
SNACKS	Time	Amount	Food Brand
LIQUIDS	Type	Amount	

EXERCISE

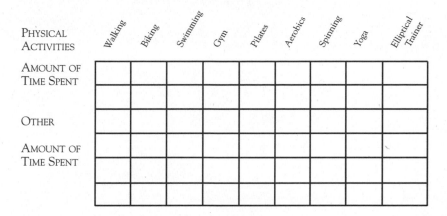

PHYSICAL ACTIVITIES	Walking	Biking	Swimming	Gym	Pilates	Aerobics	Spinning	Yoga	Elliptical Trainer
AMOUNT OF TIME SPENT									
OTHER									
AMOUNT OF TIME SPENT									

LIFESTYLE

WORK/SCHOOL	Gratifying	Satisfying	Rewarding	Exciting	Stressful	Boring	Terrible	N/A
RELATIONSHIPS	Gratifying	Satisfying	Rewarding	Exciting	Stressful	Boring	Terrible	N/A
MOOD	Good		Indifferent		Bad		Other	
SLEEP (NUMBER OF HOURS)	Continuous		Interrupted					
STRESS LEVEL (RATE 1–5)								
OVERALL RATING OF THE DAY								
(RATE 1–5)								

1=EXCELLENT

5=POOR

15

◊

In Balance:
Days 26–30

Everything I've suggested so far is easy. It's also difficult. An oxymoron? Not really. In one sense, it's not so hard to give up coffee, or soda, or cigarettes or alcohol, or sweets. In another sense, it's one of the most difficult changes you can ever go through. To change how you act in some sense changes who you are and how you think about yourself. That is what has been happening to you for the past twenty-five days.

Your life changes when your hormones are in balance. It's not a miracle—I'm not promising that you'll get married, find the perfect job, or become a millionaire just because your hormones are doing what they're supposed to do. But I am saying you'll have a better shot at reaching any goal you set for yourself. You'll have more energy to sustain you in a harsh world. You'll have the clarity to make decisions that are good for you and for those around you. You'll have the stamina and endurance you need to cope with the highs and lows that life presents. And you'll have the tools you need to deal with the inevitable stresses that are part of the human story.

These thirty days will hold you in good stead for the rest of your life. Follow the program to the best of your ability. Never beat yourself up for slipping; just pick yourself up and start all over again. Be kind to yourself while you take responsibility for creating and maintaining a healthy body—after all, it's the only one you have.

DAY 26

NATURAL HORMONES

Estradiol 0.6 mg and micronized progesterone 200 mg per day in divided doses, preferably in cream form.

DIET

- Drink water. Have at least six to eight glasses today.

- Drink at least three cups of green or other tea today.

Breakfast

Have one slice of multigrain toast and a six-ounce glass or orange or grapefruit juice. In addition, choose from:

- Oz Garcia's Favorite Smoothie (page 140).

- Three-Egg Omelet (page 164).

- Three-Egg Vegetable Omelet (follow the recipe on page 164 but add 1 cup of your favorite vegetables: steamed spinach, broccoli, mushrooms, peppers, or onions).

- 1 cup oatmeal in ½ cup skimmed milk, rice milk, or soy milk.

- Poach 2 eggs in water and pour over a plate of steamed spinach.

- 1 cup cottage cheese with a few slices of cantaloupe, apples, and/or berries, along with some granola, Total, or other high-fiber, high-protein, low-carbohydrate cereal.

- Yogurt, fruit, and granola.

○ **4 ounces cooked fish or ½ can tuna over a plate of steamed vegetables or salad greens. (Not the most popular choice for breakfast, I know, but if you like fish, give it a try!)**

Snacks

Include a snack two or three hours after both breakfast and lunch. For each snack, choose one:

○ ½ scoop Metagenics UltraClear in 1 glass of orange juice or water.

○ Protein bar.

○ Designer Whey Protein drink.

○ 2 hard-boiled eggs.

○ 1 apple, plum, or pear with 2 slices rye melba toast and tea.

○ Low-fat cottage cheese with fruit (for instance 1 cup of berries, half an apple, or half a banana).

○ 1 cup low-fat yogurt with berries and granola.

○ 10 roasted, unsalted almonds, along with 10 pieces of dried apricots, plums, or pears.

○ Cheese and crackers.

○ **1 cup soup. Homemade soups are best. If you use canned soup, be aware of the sodium content. All preserved foods have a lot of salt, and that translates into bloating and hormone imbalance; choose a low-salt variety. Vegetable soups are great as long as they are made in beef or chicken stock; otherwise they don't have enough protein to hold you over.**

Lunch and Dinner

○ Before lunch and dinner, drink an eight-ounce glass of water, and then wait ten minutes before eating.

○ At least once today, include Erika's Favorite Anytime Salad (page 142).

○ No alcoholic beverages.

○ Eliminate all soda.

○ No fast foods.

○ Reduce the number of fried or highly spiced foods you eat per week.

○ Have no more than one pasta meal or serving of potatoes for the whole week.

○ **No dessert.**

Protein Suggestions for Day 26 Lunch and Dinner

○ ¼ pound turkey breast.

○ 1 can tuna fish packed in water.

○ 1 chicken breast.

○ 1 cup tofu.

○ 8 ounces salmon, baked, grilled, or poached.

○ 8–10 pieces of sushi.

○ 6- to 8-ounce lean steak—rib or sirloin cut.

Vegetable Suggestions for Day 26 Lunch and Dinner

Have any vegetable listed under "Fiber" in chapter 5. Here are some ways to spice them up:

- 1 cup diced white or red cabbage with 3 tablespoons white vinegar and 1 tablespoon olive oil, salted to taste.

- 1 cup steamed broccoli with 1 tablespoon olive oil and a few drops of lemon, salted to taste.

- 1 cup steamed spinach with 1 tablespoon olive oil and a little salt and lemon.

- 1 cup steamed brussels sprouts with 1 tablespoon olive oil, 1 crushed garlic clove, salt, and pepper.

- ½ head steamed cabbage with 1 tablespoon olive oil, 1 crushed garlic clove, salt, and pepper.

- ½ head Boston or 2 cups romaine, red leaf, arugula, or dandelion lettuce, 1 tomato, 1 slice onion (chopped), 1 tablespoon olive oil, 1 tablespoon balsamic vinegar, salt and pepper to taste.

- 1 cup steamed beets with salt and pepper and a touch of red wine vinegar.

- 1 cup green beans steamed with 1 cup tomato sauce, ¼ teaspoon oregano, ¼ teaspoon chopped fresh dill, 1 tablespoon olive oil, 1 crushed small garlic clove, and ½ onion (diced).

- 1 cup beets, parboiled, salted, and with a drop of red wine vinegar.

- 1 cup boiled, mashed yams, flavored with nutmeg and brown sugar and baked in a 325-degree oven for 15 minutes.

- **1 cup okra (to get rid of the okra stringy things, you have to wash them in warm white wine vinegar and let them sit for 5 minutes) with tomato sauce, onions, and garlic, simmered for 10 minutes over a low flame.**

Fruit Suggestions for Day 26

Do not have more than two fruits a day, and do not eat fruit by itself before noon. Choose from:

- 1 apple.
- 1 apricot.
- 1 banana.
- ½ medium cantaloupe.
- 2 medium slices honeydew melon.
- 2 cups cherries.
- 1 medium orange.
- 2 small tangerines.
- 1 mango.
- 1 peach.
- 1 medium pear.
- 2 mandarin oranges.
- ½ cup grapes.
- 1 passion fruit.
- **1 persimmon.**

SUPPLEMENTS

Take:

- Vitamin C, 1000 mg today in the morning.
- Co Q 10, 120 mg today in the morning and at 4 P.M.

◦ Omega-3 DHA and EPA, 300 mg today in the morning and at 4 P.M.

◦ Vitamin B complex, 100 mg today in the morning.

◦ L-carnitine, 500 mg in the morning and 500 mg at 4 P.M.

◦ Calcium 1000 mg, magnesium 400 mg, and zinc 25 mg, all in one pill, in the evening before going to sleep.

EXERCISE

◦ In the morning: Start your day with ten minutes of stretching.

◦ Walk for thirty to forty-five minutes today; your pace should be a fifteen- to twenty-minute mile.

◦ Do twenty crunches: Lie with your back on the floor, your legs bent, and your feet flat on the floor. Clasp your hands behind your head. Keep your back as flat to the floor as possible. Curl your upper body forward and hold for five seconds. Don't forget to breathe.

◦ Do twenty side bends: Begin by standing up straight. Drop your head to the left. Once you feel a stretch in your neck, gently slide your left hand down your leg toward the floor. Breathe. You should feel the stretch in your right side. Hold this position for five seconds. Slowly roll back up. Repeat on the other side.

◦ Do eight to twelve biceps curls: Stand with a pair of three-pound dumbbells in your hands, palms facing front and feet shoulder width apart. Keeping your elbows stable, raise the dumbbells toward your shoulders and bring them back down slowly. You can also do this exercise while seated.

◦ **While seated, slowly raise and lower each leg in a bent position twenty times.**

◦ After dinner: If you ate out, walk for fifteen minutes before getting into your car. If that's not possible, go home and walk around your house for fifteen minutes. If you have stairs, walk up and down them for fifteen minutes.

○ If you ate at home, do not go sit on the couch as soon as you finish eating. Walk up and down two flights of stairs or around the room twenty times.

○ Do not do serious aerobic or stressful exercises after dinner; you may release adrenaline and endorphins, which will keep you awake.

○ Take ten minutes today for quiet time—meditation, personal yoga, or whatever works for you. Find a quiet place, even if it's in the bathroom. Sit down without slouching and close your eyes. Visualize something you love—a beach a forest, calming music, whatever. Then think of health permeating every cell of your body. Feel the negative energy leaving through your fingers, nose, and toes and the good energy overtaking your whole body. Start with three cleansing breaths and end with three cleansing breaths. Use this in your life whenever you feel overwhelmed, scared, or angry.

○ Include one of the following in your routine each week: a yoga, spinning, or Pilates class; a massage; or a relaxation bath or sauna.

○ **Join a gym or become part of a team activity.**

DAILY JOURNAL

Calendar Day_____

Day of Cycle_____

(Day 1 = Start of Period)

DIET

BREAKFAST	Time	Amount	Food Brand

LUNCH	Time	Amount	Food Brand

DINNER	Time	Amount	Food Brand

SNACKS	Time	Amount	Food Brand

LIQUIDS	Type	Amount

EXERCISE

PHYSICAL ACTIVITIES	Walking	Biking	Swimming	Gym	Pilates	Aerobics	Spinning	Yoga	Elliptical Trainer
AMOUNT OF TIME SPENT									
OTHER									
AMOUNT OF TIME SPENT									

LIFESTYLE

WORK/SCHOOL	Gratifying	Satisfying	Rewarding	Exciting	Stressful	Boring	Terrible	N/A
RELATIONSHIPS	Gratifying	Satisfying	Rewarding	Exciting	Stressful	Boring	Terrible	N/A
MOOD	Good		Indifferent		Bad		Other	
SLEEP (NUMBER OF HOURS)	Continuous		Interrupted					
STRESS LEVEL (RATE 1–5)								
OVERALL RATING OF THE DAY								
(RATE 1–5)								

1=EXCELLENT

5=POOR

DAY 27

NATURAL HORMONES

Same as Day 26.

DIET

- Drink water. Have at least six to eight glasses today.
- Drink at least three cups of green or other tea today.

Breakfast

Same as Day 26.

Snacks

Same as Day 26.

Lunch and Dinner

Same as Day 26.

Protein Suggestions for Day 27 Lunch and Dinner

Same as Day 26.

Vegetable Suggestions for Day 27 Lunch and Dinner

Same as Day 26.

Fruit Suggestions for Day 27

Same as Day 26.

SUPPLEMENTS

Same as Day 26.

EXERCISE

Same as Day 26.

DAILY JOURNAL

Calendar Day_____

Day of Cycle_____

(Day 1 = Start of Period)

DIET

BREAKFAST	Time	Amount	Food Brand
LUNCH	Time	Amount	Food Brand
DINNER	Time	Amount	Food Brand
SNACKS	Time	Amount	Food Brand
LIQUIDS	Type	Amount	

EXERCISE

PHYSICAL ACTIVITIES	Walking	Biking	Swimming	Gym	Pilates	Aerobics	Spinning	Yoga	Elliptical Trainer
AMOUNT OF TIME SPENT									
OTHER									
AMOUNT OF TIME SPENT									

LIFESTYLE

WORK/SCHOOL	Gratifying	Satisfying	Rewarding	Exciting	Stressful	Boring	Terrible	N/A
RELATIONSHIPS	Gratifying	Satisfying	Rewarding	Exciting	Stressful	Boring	Terrible	N/A
MOOD	Good		Indifferent		Bad		Other	
SLEEP (NUMBER OF HOURS)	Continuous		Interrupted					
STRESS LEVEL (RATE 1–5)								
OVERALL RATING OF THE DAY								
(RATE 1–5)								

1=EXCELLENT

5=POOR

DAY 28

NATURAL HORMONES

Same as Day 26.

DIET

- Drink water. Have at least six to eight glasses today.
- Drink at least three cups of green or other tea today.

Breakfast

Same as Day 26.

Snacks

Same as Day 26.

Lunch and Dinner

Same as Day 26.

Protein Suggestions for Day 28 Lunch and Dinner

Same as Day 26.

Vegetable Suggestions for Day 28 Lunch and Dinner

Same as Day 26.

Fruit Suggestions for Day 28

Same as Day 26.

SUPPLEMENTS

Same as Day 26.

EXERCISE

Same as Day 26.

DAILY JOURNAL

Calendar Day_____

Day of Cycle_____

(Day 1 = Start of Period)

DIET

BREAKFAST	Time	Amount	Food Brand
LUNCH	Time	Amount	Food Brand
DINNER	Time	Amount	Food Brand
SNACKS	Time	Amount	Food Brand
LIQUIDS	Type	Amount	

EXERCISE

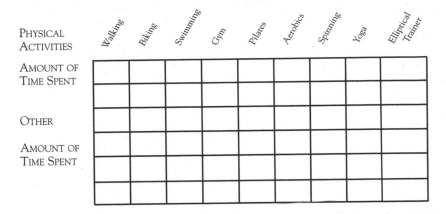

Physical Activities	Walking	Biking	Swimming	Gym	Pilates	Aerobics	Spinning	Yoga	Elliptical Trainer
Amount of Time Spent									
Other									
Amount of Time Spent									

LIFESTYLE

Work/School	Gratifying	Satisfying	Rewarding	Exciting	Stressful	Boring	Terrible	N/A
Relationships	Gratifying	Satisfying	Rewarding	Exciting	Stressful	Boring	Terrible	N/A
Mood	Good		Indifferent		Bad		Other	
Sleep (Number of Hours)	Continuous		Interrupted					
Stress Level (Rate 1–5)								
Overall Rating of the Day (Rate 1–5)								

1=Excellent

5=Poor

DAY 29

NATURAL HORMONES

Same as Day 26.

DIET

○ Drink water. Have at least six to eight glasses today.
○ Drink at least three cups of green or other tea today.

Breakfast

Same as Day 26.

Snacks

Same as Day 26.

Lunch and Dinner

Same as Day 26.

Protein Suggestions for Day 29 Lunch and Dinner

Same as Day 26.

Vegetable Suggestions for Day 29 Lunch and Dinner

Same as Day 26.

Fruit Suggestions for Day 29

Same as Day 26.

SUPPLEMENTS

Same as Day 26.

EXERCISE

Same as Day 26.

DAILY JOURNAL

Calendar Day_____

Day of Cycle_____

(Day 1 = Start of Period)

DIET

BREAKFAST	Time	Amount	Food Brand

LUNCH	Time	Amount	Food Brand

DINNER	Time	Amount	Food Brand

SNACKS	Time	Amount	Food Brand

LIQUIDS	Type	Amount	

EXERCISE

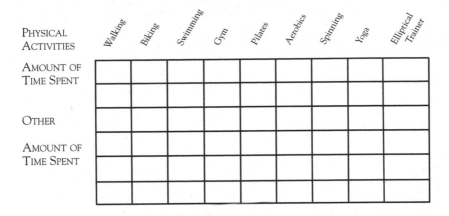

PHYSICAL ACTIVITIES	Walking	Biking	Swimming	Gym	Pilates	Aerobics	Spinning	Yoga	Elliptical Trainer
AMOUNT OF TIME SPENT									
OTHER									
AMOUNT OF TIME SPENT									

LIFESTYLE

WORK/SCHOOL	Gratifying	Satisfying	Rewarding	Exciting	Stressful	Boring	Terrible	N/A
RELATIONSHIPS	Gratifying	Satisfying	Rewarding	Exciting	Stressful	Boring	Terrible	N/A
MOOD	Good		Indifferent		Bad		Other	
SLEEP (NUMBER OF HOURS)	Continuous		Interrupted					
STRESS LEVEL (RATE 1–5)								
OVERALL RATING OF THE DAY								
(RATE 1–5)								

1=EXCELLENT

5=POOR

DAY 30

NATURAL HORMONES

Same as Day 26.

DIET

- Drink water. Have at least six to eight glasses today.
- Drink at least three cups of green or other tea today.

Breakfast

Same as Day 26.

Snacks

Same as Day 26.

Lunch and Dinner

Same as Day 26.

Protein Suggestions for Day 30 Lunch and Dinner

Same as Day 26.

Vegetable Suggestions for Day 30 Lunch and Dinner

Same as Day 26.

Fruit Suggestions for Day 30

Same as Day 26.

SUPPLEMENTS

Same as Day 26.

EXERCISE

Same as Day 26.

DAILY JOURNAL

Calendar Day_____

Day of Cycle_____

(Day 1 = Start of Period)

DIET

BREAKFAST	Time	Amount	Food Brand
LUNCH	Time	Amount	Food Brand
DINNER	Time	Amount	Food Brand
SNACKS	Time	Amount	Food Brand
LIQUIDS	Type	Amount	

EXERCISE

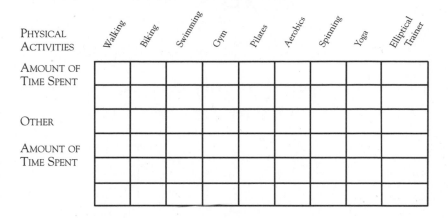

Physical Activities	Walking	Biking	Swimming	Gym	Pilates	Aerobics	Spinning	Yoga	Elliptical Trainer
Amount of Time Spent									
Other									
Amount of Time Spent									

LIFESTYLE

Work/School	Gratifying	Satisfying	Rewarding	Exciting	Stressful	Boring	Terrible	N/A
Relationships	Gratifying	Satisfying	Rewarding	Exciting	Stressful	Boring	Terrible	N/A
Mood	Good		Indifferent		Bad		Other	
Sleep (Number of Hours)	Continuous		Interrupted					
Stress Level (Rate 1–5)								
Overall Rating of the Day								
(Rate 1–5)								

1=Excellent

5=Poor

16

◯

Hormone-Friendly Recipes, Part 2

Here are some more recipes for you to enjoy. They contain hormone-friendly ingredients, are easy to make, and will add some variety into your lunches and dinners. Your diet does not have to be bland or boring to be healthy, and these recipes will prove it!

All-Season Vegetable Combo Costel

3 tablespoons olive oil
1 medium onion, chopped
1 cauliflower, in chunks
1 parsnip, chopped
10 small carrots or 2 large carrots, chopped
2 medium Idaho potatoes, cubed
1 cup halved string beans
½ cup green peas
1 small eggplant, cubed
¼ bunch Italian parsley
2 cups hot water with two chicken bouillon cubes dissolved
1 can tomato paste
3 large tomatoes, cubed, or 10 cherry tomatoes or 5 plum tomatoes, halved
salt to taste

Heat the olive oil with the chopped onion in a stew pot over high flame until the onion is golden brown. Add all the vegetables (except the tomatoes), along with the water and bouillon cubes, and cover. Simmer for 10 minutes.

Transfer into a baking pan. Place in 325-degree oven, adding the tomato paste and enough extra water to dilute the paste and cover the vegetables. After 15 to 20 minutes, place the tomatoes on top of the vegetables and bake for another 20 minutes. Salt to taste and serve either hot or cold.

6 SERVINGS

Winter Vegetable Chicken Lisa

3 tablespoons olive oil
2 garlic cloves, chopped
1 medium onion, chopped
1 chicken breast, cut into 1-inch thick slices
rock salt
1 small can tomato paste thinned with 1 cup warm water
1 medium Idaho potato, cubed
½ bunch Italian parsley
3 small carrots
1 parsnip
1 green pepper, chopped
¼ cup green peas
2 large tomatoes in round slices ½ inch thick
1 glass white wine
salt
pepper

Heat the oil in a stew pot. Add the garlic and brown it. Add the onion and brown. Rub the chicken with rock salt and add to the pot. Stir-fry for 5 minutes. Add the tomato paste and water. Add the potato and half of the parsley. Cover and simmer for 10 minutes. Place

the chicken, potato, and sauce on a deep baking sheet and add
the remaining vegetables (except the tomatoes) and parsley. Place the
tomatoes on top, cover with aluminum foil, and bake in a 325-degree
oven for 20 minutes. Sprinkle with wine and leave uncovered in the
oven for 3 minutes. Salt and pepper to taste, and serve hot.

4 SERVINGS

Variation: This recipe can also be made with beef sirloin, turkey
breast, veal, or salmon instead of chicken.

Winter Beef with White Beans Sylvia

> 3 tablespoons olive oil
> 1 medium onion, chopped
> 1 pound sirloin, cubed
> 1 can tomato paste thinned with 1 cup warm water
> 1 bay leaf
> 1 pound white beans
> ½ bunch Italian parsley
> salt
> pepper

Heat the oil in stew pot and add the onion to brown. Add the beef.
Stir-fry for 5 minutes. Add the tomato paste and water and bay leaf.
    Put the white beans in a separate pot, add cold water to cover,
and boil over a medium to high flame. After they are 30 percent
cooked (medium hard), discard the water and replace it with fresh
boiling water. When the beans are fully cooked, add them to the
meat along with the parsley. Continue cooking till fully cooked.
Salt and pepper to taste, and serve hot.

4 SERVINGS

Variation: This recipe can also be made with chicken or monkfish
instead of beef.

Sesame Chicken Sharyn

4 chicken thighs and legs
rock salt
3 tablespoons olive oil
3 tablespoons sesame seeds
½ cup lite soy sauce

Soak the chicken legs and thighs overnight in rock salt brine. Dry, then coat with olive oil and roll in sesame seeds. Place on a cookie sheet or shallow baking pan and sprinkle with soy sauce. Bake at 350 degrees for 1 hour or until fully cooked.

3–4 SERVINGS

Shrimp in Lemon Sauce Carmela

3 tablespoons olive oil
½ cup freshly squeezed lemon juice
½ glass white wine
1 garlic clove, chopped
salt and pepper
1 pound cleaned medium or large shrimp
½ bunch parsley

In a large skillet slowly heat the olive oil, lemon juice, and wine. Simmer for 5 minutes; when thoroughly hot, stir in the garlic, pepper, and salt. Mix constantly. Reduce the heat to medium and add the shrimp while tossing continuously. Cook for 5 minutes until cooked (they should be light pink). Add the parsley before serving. Serve immediately with 1 cup basmati rice.

2 SERVINGS

Weekly Pasta Dish Maria

3 tablespoons oil
2 garlic cloves, sliced thin
1 pound pasta (any type you desire)
salt and pepper to taste

In a small frying pan, heat 2 tablespoons of olive oil over a high flame. Add the garlic and sauté till light brown and crispy. Cook the pasta al dente. Rinse with cold water once and fresh hot water immediately afterward. Toss with the remaining 1 tablespoon of olive oil, warmed, then add the garlic with oil and salt and pepper to taste. Serve immediately.

4 SERVINGS

The Best Lunch Chicken Salad Odette

½ head romaine lettuce, cut in bite-size pieces
1 large tomato, cubed, or 3 cherry tomatoes
½ avocado, sliced
2 radishes, sliced
2 small carrots, slivered
1 small onion, sliced (optional)
2 tablespoons olive oil
salt and pepper to taste
1 teaspoon red wine vinegar
2 tablespoons lemon juice
1 chicken breast, skinned, roasted, and sliced in 1-inch slices

Toss all the ingredients except the chicken with the oil, salt, vinegar, and lemon juice. Season the chicken with salt and pepper and a drop of oil. Place the salad in a serving dish and add chicken slices on top.

1 SERVING

Sole Marinade Ken

1 pound sole
2 tablespoons flour
salt
pepper
3 tablespoons oil
2 tablespoons red wine vinegar
2 tablespoons tomato paste
2 bay leaves

Lightly flour the sole and place it in a baking pan; add pepper and salt. Sprinkle with the olive oil and red wine vinegar. Cover with the tomato paste and ½ cup warm water and add bay leaves. Bake in a 350-degree oven for 15 minutes covered with aluminum foil. Remove the foil and bake for an additional 5 minutes. Serve warm.

2 SERVINGS

Tomato Cabbage Olivia

1 white cabbage, chopped
3 tablespoons tomato paste
4 small tomatoes
½ cup chicken or vegetable broth
1 green pepper, chopped
3 tablespoons olive oil
salt

Place the cabbage flat in a baking dish. Add all the remaining ingredients, sprinkling them finely over the cabbage. Cover with aluminum foil and place in a 325-degree oven. Bake for 25 minutes. Remove the foil and bake for another 5 minutes. Serve either cold or hot.

2 SERVINGS

Vegetable Soup Deborah

1 large carrot
1 bunch Italian parsley
1 small parsnip
1 medium onion
½ small cabbage
1 small head Boston lettuce
2 leeks
salt
¼ teaspoon brown sugar
2 tablespoons olive oil
6 cups broth, vegetable or chicken

Dice all the vegetables thinly, like spaghetti. Mix in a bowl. Add the salt and sugar. Place in a stew pot with olive oil, cover, and simmer for 5 minutes. Mix gently with a wooden spoon. Add the broth. Cook for 20 minutes. Serve warm.

4 SERVINGS

Odette's Tomato Soup

½ shallot
½ tablespoon olive oil
1 celery stalk, finely chopped
1 8-ounce can stewed tomatoes
1 can lite chicken broth
salt
½ cup tightly packed chopped fresh basil

Sauté the shallot in the oil and add the celery. Cook for 5 minutes until the vegetables are soft. Add all the remaining ingredients except the basil. Simmer for 15 minutes. Puree in the blender and rewarm. Serve with basil garnish.

2–3 SERVINGS

Carrot Soup Brendan

1 pound large carrots
2 tablespoons olive oil
1 medium onion, chopped
salt
½ teaspoon brown sugar
4 large potatoes, peeled and thinly sliced
6 cups water or broth

Cut the carrots into thin slices. Place them in a pot with the olive oil and simmer with the onion. When the carrots get soft, add the salt, sugar, and potatoes. Add the liquid. Cover and let cook over medium heat for 30 minutes. Puree and serve.

4 SERVINGS

Peas with Lemon Katie

1 pound green peas
2 tablespoons olive oil
juice and grated rind of 1 lemon
salt

In pot ⅓ filled with salted water at the boiling point, add the peas and cook for 5 minutes or until bright green. Drain and place in cold water. Add the olive oil to a skillet, then add the peas and toss for 3 minutes. Remove the peas and place them in a bowl with the lemon juice, lemon rind, and salt. Toss and serve.

4 SERVINGS

Roasted Sliced Fennel Bulb Elissa

1 fennel bulb, trimmed, with tops and outside leaves removed, cut lengthwise into ¼-inch-thick slices
3 tablespoons olive oil
1 tablespoon fresh lemon juice
rock salt and pepper to taste

In an oven preheated to 500 degrees, place the fennel slices on a cookie sheet on the bottom rack. Sprinkle some of the olive oil on the slices. Keep them in one layer. Turn after 15 minutes and roast for another 15 minutes. Sprinkle with the remaining olive oil, lemon juice, salt, and pepper. Serve hot or cold.

2 SERVINGS

Damon's Steamed Fish with Ginger

4 fish fillets (flaky fish is best)
4 green onions, finely diced
3 tablespoons grated fresh ginger
3 tablespoons lite soy sauce
2 teaspoons grated lemon zest

Place the fish on a heatproof plate on a steamer rack. In a small bowl, mix the green onions, ginger, soy sauce, and zest. Spread this mixture on top of the fish. Boil water in the steamer pot underneath. Cover and steam until fish is cooked—10 minutes for thin fillets, 15 for thicker. Serve hot.

4 SERVINGS

Cucumber Salad Caroline

2 tablespoons plus two teaspoons brown sugar
⅓ teaspoon salt
2 tablespoons white vinegar
10 ¼-inch-thick cucumber slices, cut up
4–5 thin slices red onion, diced
3–4 round slices jalapeño pepper, chopped
3 sprigs coriander, chopped

Combine the sugar, salt, and vinegar in a small saucepan to make a sweet-and-sour sauce. Heat over a medium flame, stirring, until all the ingredients are dissolved. Cool. Mix the cucumbers, red onion, and pepper in a small bowl. Add the sweet-and-sour sauce and coriander. Serve cool.

2 SERVINGS

Eggplant Dip Jasper

1 large eggplant
3 tablespoons olive oil
½ lemon, juiced
1 garlic clove, mashed
salt and pepper to taste

Grill the eggplant on aluminum foil on a cooktop until soft on all sides. Clean the skin off and drain any excess water from the pulp. Add the oil, lemon, garlic, salt, and pepper. Mix with a fork or egg beater until frothy. Serve with toasted pita bread.

4 SERVINGS

Avocado Corn Salsa Amy

1 cup cooked corn
¼ cup chopped red bell pepper
¼ cup chopped yellow bell pepper
¼ cup diced tomatoes
2 tablespoons chopped fresh cilantro
salt and pepper to taste
2 tablespoons lemon juice
1 tablespoon shallots, finely chopped
½ jalapeño pepper, seeded and chopped
Mexican hot sauce to taste
1 cup diced avocado

Mix all the ingredients except the avocado and chill. Add the avocado just before serving. Mix and serve with tortilla chips.

3–4 SERVINGS

Honey-Orange Chicken Alex

1 egg
1 teaspoon water
½ cup matzo meal or bread crumbs
salt and pepper to taste
1 cut-up chicken
3 tablespoons olive oil
½ cup hot water
2 tablespoons honey
½ cup orange juice

Beat the egg with the water. Mix the crumbs with salt and pepper. Dip the chicken in the egg mixture, then coat with the crumb mixture. Place in a skillet with the oil and brown for 5 minutes. Remove and drain. Mix the hot water with the honey and orange juice. Place the chicken in a 325-degree oven and cover with sauce. Bake for 45 minutes, uncovered, basting occasionally.

3 SERVINGS

Chicken with Lime Bethany

3 tablespoons lime juice
½ tablespoon Worcestershire or lite soy sauce
1 teaspoon crushed garlic
1 teaspoon dry mustard
12 boneless chicken breasts
pepper and salt to taste

Mix the lime with the Worcestershire sauce, garlic, and mustard. Marinate the chicken in this mixture for 30 minutes. Remove, sprinkle with pepper and salt, and place on the grill or in the broiler for 7 minutes on each side. Serve hot or cold.

6 SERVINGS

Salmon and Arugula Salad Wendy

1 pound fresh salmon
sea salt
1 pound fresh arugula
2 medium tomatoes (or 5 cherry tomatoes)
2 tablespoons olive oil
1 tablespoon red wine vinegar
salt and pepper to taste

Rub salmon with sea salt and let sit for 10 minutes. Place in 350-degree preheated oven. Cook for 20 minutes or until flaky and moist. Prepare arugula: Wash thoroughly, spin dry, and cut into small pieces, removing stems. Cut tomatoes into cubes. Toss with oil, vinegar, salt, and pepper. Serve salmon on top of arugula salad.

2–3 SERVINGS

17

◯

And Life Goes On . . .
Special Situations and
Lifelong Maintenance

FALLING OFF THE
HORMONAL WAGON

I tell my patients all the time: "Remember, above all, you are human!" The human body is a beautiful dynamic system. Its internal balance changes all the time. Understanding how you function should lower expectations about your ability to stay on any given program with unwavering tenacity. When you have reasonable expectations, you can enjoy the occasional ice cream, martini, or large helping of pasta without feeling guilty or falling off the wagon for weeks.

෴

Maryanne is forty-eight. Balancing her hormones was a difficult task. Her personal and professional lives were in turmoil. Within six months, she had gone through a divorce and a job change. Along came hot flashes, night sweats, and dreaded palpitations every morning at 5 A.M. She underwent thorough examinations and heart evaluations, and no abnormalities were found. To help her find relief from her symptoms, I started her on natural hormones and supplements and placed her on a very intensive version of the 30-Day Plan involving follow-up with me every two weeks.

Maryanne found the first two weeks difficult. She could not live without four cups of coffee a day. Needless to say, although slightly improved, many of her symptoms persisted. Finally, Maryanne realized that she would feel better if she followed the whole program; she decided to eliminate the coffee, and as a result felt remarkably improved. We agreed that she should come see me again in six months.

Three months later, I received a panicked phone call from Maryanne. She had done very well for the first thirty days of the program. But something went awry two months later, and her hot flashes had returned; in addition, she was experiencing palpitations every morning again. Before I could ask, Maryanne told me that she'd had to move, and the stress was too much to bear. I asked her to come see me. She agreed but did not show up for the appointment. When I called her, she told me she had forgotten and had to put going back on the program on hold because of time constraints.

Two months later, Maryanne called me again. This time she was in even worse shape. She had gained ten pounds, was drinking coffee again, was seriously depressed, had started to forget things, and all her symptoms had returned. This time she did come in to see me. She told me that she realized the only way to feel better again—to regain control over her life—would be to make the time for herself and recommit to the 30-Day Plan. She did just that. Two weeks later, Maryanne felt so much better that she called to volunteer to become a testimonial to the program. Three years later, Maryanne has joined our team of educators. She gives lectures to women's groups and uses her own personal experience to motivate other women in search of hormone balance and improvement in their quality of life.

❧

Maryanne is typical of the patients I work with. She is human and lives an often difficult but always real life. I like working with people like Maryanne, because they invariably do well on the program. They learn firsthand how their bodies work. Once they experience the difference in their bodies between being on the program and not, they are less likely to completely fall off the wagon again.

EVERYDAY CHALLENGES: EATING OUT

It doesn't always take unusual stress or trauma to throw us off our game. Everyday occurrences can present challenges as well. One of the most challenging situations is eating healthy while eating out.

The hormone-friendly diet program I outlined is easy to follow when you eat at home. But in today's hectic world, many of us find restaurant dining (whether we eat in or take out) a large part of our lives. There are several drawbacks to going out to dinner: You don't always know exactly what you're eating. You're not in control of the ingredients placed in your food. In America, portions have become gigantic—and we've all been taught to eat whatever is on our plates, so we do. Not the ideal situation for anyone trying to follow a program of moderation and balance to benefit hormones or general health.

So how do we enjoy going out to dinner while still benefiting from following the general guidelines of the 30-Day Plan?

Simply remember the basic *No-nos* of the diet and follow them when you go out.

- No coffee.
- No soda.
- Little or no alcohol.
- No spicy foods.
- No overeating.
- No dessert.
- No eating after 8:30 P.M.

Most restaurants have a variety of dishes on the menu—some healthier than others. Try to follow the guidelines of the 30-Day Plan. If you want to "pig out" every once in a while, go for it. But most times, choose something simple. Tell the waiter how you'd like your dish prepared—but don't be so obsessive that you can't enjoy yourself and your meal.

HEALTHY-HORMONE CHOICES FOR ETHNIC FARE

Following is a list of the most popular types of restaurants and some of the foods they serve, divided into hormone-friendly and -unfriendly categories. Use them as guidelines when you go out.

ITALIAN FOOD

Hormone Friendly

- Minestrone.
- Seafood soup.
- Straciatella soup.
- Mussels marinara.
- Pasta with marinara sauce.
- Pasta primavera.
- Bread sticks without butter.
- Veal piccata or Marsala.
- Seafood dishes (not fried).
- Steamed vegetable side dishes.

Hormone Unfriendly

- Antipasto.
- Garlic bread.
- Fettuccine Alfredo.
- Parmigiana dishes.
- Meat sauces.
- Lasagna.
- Cannelloni.
- Gelato.
- All desserts.

MEXICAN FOOD

Hormone Friendly

• Black bean soup.
• Gazpacho.
• Ceviche (marinated fish).
• Nopalitos (baby cactus salad).
• Salsa.
• Grilled chicken or shrimp.
• Stewed seafood dishes.
• Fajitas (without the sour cream).
• Corn or wheat tortillas.
• Guacamole.

Hormone Unfriendly

• Nachos.
• Flautas.
• Tortilla chips.
• Refried beans.
• Chimichangas.
• Sour cream.
• Enchiladas.
• Fried flour tortillas.

JAPANESE FOOD

Hormone Friendly

• Miso soup.
• Sushi.
• Sashimi.
• Teriyaki.
• Oshinko (pickled vegetables).

- Yakitori (broiled chicken).
- Yakimono (boiled fish or chicken).
- Maki rolls.
- Steamed tofu.
- Shabu-shabu (boiled meat, seafood, and vegetables).

Hormone Unfriendly

- Tempura.
- Tonkatsu (fried pork).
- Torikatsu (fried chicken).
- Age tofu (fried tofu).
- Fried ice cream.

Remember that soy sauce is high in sodium; ask for reduced-sodium soy sauce, or dilute with water.

INDIAN FOOD

Hormone Friendly

- Dal (lentils).
- Mulligatawny soup (lentils).
- Mango chutney.
- Sweet-and-sour cabbage.
- Vegetable curries.
- Dal palak (split peas).
- Nan (baked bread).
- Pulka (unleavened bread).
- Basmati rice with vegetables.
- Tandoori chicken or fish.
- Biryanis (rice dish).

Hormone Unfriendly

- Puri (fried bread).
- Coconut milk curry sauces.
- Samosa (fried appetizers).
- Muglai (creamy curry sauce).

DINNER AT MIDNIGHT, TRAVEL, AND OTHER TRANSITIONAL CHALLENGES

It's not always easy to keep to your schedule and maintain your new healthy habits. When you travel, it's even harder. Temptations abound. We tend to eat three large meals a day on the road, and have dinner a lot later than we do at home.

Although a moonlit midnight meal may be good for romance, it's not so good for your health. Hormones are made during the night. When you eat late in the evening, your body has to focus all its resources on digesting the meal. Your hormones and digestive enzymes have to break down the foodstuffs into usable energy and store what's left over. This is a complex and lengthy process that requires energy and time and detracts from the processes needed to make hormones.

Unless you come from a culture where dining late is the norm, the wear and tear on your body caused by a midnight meal doesn't really justify its romantic appeal.

Even if you forgo the midnight meals, travel imparts significant wear and tear to our bodies. Data have emerged on the increased frequency of short-term illnesses such as flu and colds associated with travel in general, and air travel in particular.

No matter what the mode of transportation, travel poses hazards to your physiology. Trying to maintain balance in a constantly changing environment is difficult. We must identify the potential problems associated with travel and then develop easy, user-friendly ways of preventing the damage from occurring.

Sitting for prolonged periods of time compromises hormone balance and increases blood thickness. The mechanism that causes this change in blood consistency is not well understood, but the outcome is known to be dangerous: increased risk of blood clots and phlebitis. This is less likely with train travel, because people move around more on trains. Risk reduction involves being aware of the potential problem and moving as much as possible.

- Stand up and stretch every two hours.
- Tighten your calf muscles ten times every two hours.
- Rotate your feet clockwise and counterclockwise ten times every two hours.
- Tighten your buttocks and count to ten.
- Push your shoulder blades back and down as far as possible and try to have them meet in the middle of your back.
- Cock your head and stretch your neck. (Do not push your head forward; push it up.)
- Stretch your arms to the ceiling and pull your whole body up like a marionette.
- Clasp your hands together and, reaching over your head, try to touch the middle of your back.

Another problem is that, although most airlines will deny it, recirculated air on planes is not as clean as you might like it to be. The longer the flight, the more likely you are to be exposed to the risk of catching a cold from other passengers on board. There's not much you can do about the actual flying time. It's pretty much the same situation as when you work in close quarters with other people for a prolonged period of time. But you can protect yourself by following the 30-Day Plan at all times: eating well, getting enough rest before and after the trip, staying away from immune busters such as alcohol and coffee, and maintaining your exercise program.

Once you reach your destination, maintain a reasonable schedule whenever possible. Get seven to eight hours of sleep a night, drink six to ten glasses of water a day, eat foods that are similar in composition to those you eat at home, and preserve a consistent level of physical activity or exercise program. Inertia is a most dangerous habit. When you stop exercising or moving, your body gets lazy and will perpetuate the lack of motion, which translates into aging and physical deterioration secondary to hormone depletion: a deadly combination.

Indeed, one of the most difficult elements of the program to maintain is the exercise portion. Whether you travel on business or are on vacation and find running to the gym or the swimming pool too difficult to fit into your schedule, try my simple exercise routine in your room. It doesn't add stress, it takes ten minutes, and it helps keep your hormones in balance, your body limber and strong, and your metabolic rate up.

- Every morning before taking a shower or leaving your room, get on the floor and do thirty sit-ups while watching the morning news on TV or planning the day ahead.
- Do thirty side bends (see page 197).
- Get two bottles of mineral water, one liter each, and use them as weights for biceps curls. Pump them in repetitions of ten. Do it three times after finishing your sit-ups (see page 248).
- Place your back flush against the wall, your feet flat on the floor. Slide into a sitting position (with your back still against the wall). Hold for one minute.
- Stretch for two minutes.
- Sit on the floor and cradle your knees to your chest. Hold for one minute.
- Run in place for two minutes.

JET LAG AND SLEEP DEPRIVATION

From 1994 to 1999, I served as medical consultant to KLM Royal Dutch Airlines. In this capacity, I was involved with various medical issues related to air travel. Jet lag and sleep deprivation created significant discomfort for most passengers and airline staff and have become chronic quandaries of the twenty-first-century traveler.

Jet lag is a sleep deprivation reaction associated with changes in time zones. Research in the etiology and treatment of jet lag has found no consistent solutions to the problem. For a while, the hormone melatonin appeared to be the answer; unfortunately, bona fide medical research failed to support these claims, and slowly travelers shied away from yet another disappointing wishful cure.

Humans are hormonally built to stay in one time zone and get a restful seven to eight hours of sleep a night. When we don't get the rest, and especially when we travel east to west, the hormone balance gets disrupted and results in jet lag. To some people, this means walking around in brain fog for days; for others, it's a generalized malaise that affects their thinking as well as their appetite and sense of well-being. As we age, jet lag lasts longer and becomes even more disruptive and of longer duration. So what should you do? Stop traveling?

While you may not be able to totally eliminate its nefarious effects, there are things you can do to protect your hormone balance and improve your chances of surviving jet lag with minimal hormonal inconvenience. Prepare. Two weeks before you travel, start with Weeks 3 and 4 of the 30-Day Plan. If that's not an option, follow the following ground rules:

- Get plenty of rest forty-eight hours before going on the flight. Try to sleep at least eight hours for a couple of nights before you fly.
- The day before you fly, get into the time zone schedule you are going to. For instance, if you go to Europe, move your day six hours ahead and live as though you are six hours ahead.
- Drink lots of water.
- Do not drink any alcohol for three days before you fly or during the flight.
- Do not drink coffee or other stimulants when you arrive at your destination.
- Take a two-hour nap when you arrive at your destination if you can.

• Sleep on the plane rather than watching movies or reading.
• Do not work on the plane.

Your body will adjust in time. Be patient and accept the transition. Stay on the 30-Day Plan to make your journey, and your adjustment, easier.

PART IV

THE POLITICS OF HORMONES

18

◯

Synthetic Suicide:
The National Institutes of Health/Women's
Health Initiative Study and Its Aftermath

Until seventy-five years ago, medications were prepared as per doctor's orders by pharmacists who personally mixed the ingredients together for the individual patient. Medications consisted of salves, ointments, powders, and syrups derived mostly from plants.

Because they were not standardized (meaning the same dose and makeup every time), the patient received a slightly different medication every time. The medication's effectiveness was not tested thoroughly through clinical or laboratory studies. Treatment was given one person at a time. Medicine was even more an art than a science.

That was before pharmaceutical companies entered the market. Pharmaceutical companies began to appear in the 1930s, first in Europe and soon after in the United States. To make medications in large quantities available to large numbers of people, the first step was to introduce standardization into the industry. This innovation allowed mass production as well as the commercialization of pharmaceutical products.

As the pharmaceutical industry expanded, it focused on developing new drugs. Antibiotics were the first mass-produced medications; vaccines followed soon after. Without pharmaceuticals, we would not have conquered infectious diseases or prevented epidemics from spreading and killing millions of people.

Pharmaceuticals are saviors to millions of people every day. Part of the credit for our increased life expectancy goes to advances made through contributions by the pharmaceutical industry. But as with every great positive, there is a dark side to pharmaceuticals. Success breeds greed, and the pharmaceutical industry has not been spared its share. Remember, pharmaceutical medications originally all came from natural sources. As the industry evolved, a major change in the source of medications occurred. The invention of synthetic medications exploded the industry.

Synthetic medications are human-made or human-altered products. They have unique molecular formulations that do not exist in nature. As discussed in chapter 3, this uniqueness translates into patentability, thus proprietorship. Proprietary medications and the astronomical revenues they bring have allowed the pharmaceutical industry to become the most powerful force in the economics of health care. The process by which pharmaceutical companies have accomplished this immense feat is simple to understand and brilliant in its strategy.

The Food and Drug Administration, the governmental agency that oversees the safety and efficacy of pharmaceutical products, was initially developed in response to the aggressive marketing and development of products by the pharmaceutical industry. The FDA has to approve medications before they can be mass-marketed in the United States. This approval process is lengthy (years) and expensive (multi-million dollars per drug). Only a wealthy industry can participate in such a process, and its financial rewards must be commensurate to the investment. This means that competition in any drug must be limited or eliminated.

The only guaranteed protection against competition is offered through patents. Patent protection secures the investment and, if the drug becomes popular, guarantees financial reward. The problem is that only medications with new (in other words, "unique," "novel," and "non-obvious") chemical formulations that cannot be found in nature can be granted patents. If a drug does not qualify for a patent (for instance, an herbal or otherwise naturally occurring substance), other pharmaceutical companies can also manufacture and sell it. To avoid the loss of income produced by lack of patent protection, pharmaceutical companies have in the past twenty-five years focused exclusively on the development of synthetic drugs.

Therefore, unfortunately, drugs with chemical structures found in nature (such as natural hormones—estradiol, estriol, estrone, micronized progesterone)—medications with potentially great value to the public—have been ignored by pharmaceutical companies in their frenzy to protect their financial investments.

THE SAGA OF SYNTHETIC HORMONE REPLACEMENT THERAPY

For the above reasons, pharmaceutical companies have stayed away from natural hormones. Since natural hormones are bioidentical, meaning they have the same chemical formula as our bodies' own hormones and are made from soy and yam oils (natural sources), they cannot be patented. From a purely economic standpoint, natural hormones are undesirable to the pharmaceutical industry. They are not worth the financial investment of testing and promoting them.

The result is that we are now faced with a terrible situation caused by fifty years of synthetic hormone replacement therapies and forty years of birth control pills that have left behind serious medical problems, questions of safety, confusion about hormones in general, and potentially significant health hazards.

Since its arrival on the market in the late 1950s, HRT has been synonymous with synthetics. Neither physicians nor members of the public are clearly aware of the fundamental distinction between synthetic hormones and hormones in general—the hormones made by our bodies. All large-scale, well-funded, highly publicized studies on the efficacy, safety, and long-term effect of HRT have been conducted exclusively on synthetic hormones. Because of the vast and expensive marketing and education efforts by pharmaceutical companies, most people, physicians included, have made the incorrect assumption that synthetic hormones are the only viable form of hormone replacement available.

Behind the scenes, however, and away from the public eye, natural hormones received FDA approval many years ago. To obtain this approval, they had to follow the same rigid criteria followed by their synthetic counterparts. Since then, natural hormones have been extensively studied, and used by physicians, scientists, and women who found them helpful and safe. Still, the visibility of these studies, which lacked major governmental support and funding, has remained low.

The movement against synthetic hormone replacement therapy has been brewing for many years. A seminal article in the May 1994 *American Journal of Obstetrics and Gynecology* by J. D. Woodruff and J. H. Pickar established that synthetic estrogen replacement therapy (specifically Premarin) was associated with an increased incidence of endometrial hyperplasia, which is an increased thickness of the lining of the uterus and is often a precursor to uterine cancer. It was a seminal article to raise the issue of dangerous side effects from synthetic HRT, but it certainly was not to be the last.

In 1994, the National Institutes of Health (NIH), fully funded by the pharmaceutical manufacturers of HRT (Wyeth, producers of Premarin and Prempro) and hundreds of academic medical centers across the United States, started an enormous study on the long-term effects of synthetic hormones on menopausal women's health. The study, titled the Women's Health Initiative, involved more than twenty-five thousand menopausal women. It was supposed to follow them for eight and a half years and look at the long-term effects of synthetic hormone replacement therapy (Premarin and Prempro) in the prevention of heart disease, osteoporosis, cancer, and Alzheimer's disease.

Going into the study, the claims made on behalf of synthetic HRT were that the drugs were designed to provide cardiac protection, and also helped prevent osteoporosis and certain types of cancers. These claims were not based on definitive scientific data or results of long-term, large-scale clinical research, but rather on the manufacturer's hypothesis stemming from small observational surveys and, as one of the principal investigators, Dr. Susan Hendrix of Wayne State University, stated, a "hypothesis made by the Women's Health Initiative investigators."

If anyone but the prestigious National Institutes of Health had tried to conduct a study with such flimsy data supporting it, I don't believe that it would have been able to do it.

The NIH study was designed to follow the most stringent protocols. Hundreds of millions of dollars were spent on formatting and implementing this study. Two years into the study, however, troubling data emerged:

HRT AND CARDIOVASCULAR EVENTS: WHI PRELIMINARY RESULTS

- After 2 years, following trends identified:
  —Increase in cardiovascular events (MI, stroke, VTE) in
     HRT groups vs placebo
  —Risk perhaps higher with addition of progestin
  —Trend expected to diminish over time

NIH Press Release, April 3, 2000.

As the above press release by the National Institutes of Health in April 2000 noted, the risks of heart attacks and strokes appeared to be increased in the participants in the study taking HRT. Still, the NIH allowed the study to continue, evidently "hoping" the trend would diminish over time.

More than five years into the study, on July 9, 2002, one arm of the Women's Health Initiative was abruptly stopped with an enormous amount of fanfare and media coverage. These were the reasons given:

WHI STUDY HALTED

- On July 9, 2002 at 5.2 years
- Risks outweighed the benefits
- Increased risks of:
  - Breast cancer
  - CHD
  - Stroke
  - Blood clots

Unbelievably, another arm of the study, involving ten thousand women (of whom at least half are taking Premarin) without uteruses (that is, posthysterectomy) continues. Amid controversy and valid, duplicated scientific data going back almost twenty years connecting treatment with synthetic hormones to potentially deadly side effects, the study continues. The question in my mind is, Why? And why are we not looking at other, potentially safer options instead of beating a dead horse into the ground?

The halted study of the Women's Health Initiative has left the medical community without adequate direction for the treatment of menopause and hormone imbalances, and the public desperate for answers and solutions. Synthetic hormones have been dealt a near-fatal blow, with a long-lasting impact on how hormone therapy seems to be perceived in general.

Because the Women's Health Initiative was limited in its scope and studied only synthetic hormones, it left a gaping hole in information and education on natural hormones. Although natural hormones have not suffered directly from the failed study (because they were not part of the trials), they have been affected indirectly. Before July 9, 2002, natural hormones were out of the limelight, their use limited to a few expert physicians who were treating a select few fortunate patients. As recently as five years ago, most conventional physicians didn't even know they existed as a conventional medicine option, even though they are a prescription medication and FDA approved.

As more baby boomers entered menopause and became interested in other nonsynthetic options for treatment of symptoms, a growing information gap developed between the public and the medical profession. As the public turned toward alternative options—synthetic hormones and *natural* treatments—many women *discovered natural hormones, found the doctors who would prescribe them, and, satisfied with the results, created increasing demand for them.*

Unfortunately, the medical profession has been in no position to accommodate this growing need. Lacking the necessary education, usually generated through the pharmaceutical companies, scientific data, and general knowledge, to meet the public demand for natural hormones, conventional medicine has been stuck precribing synthetic HRT—and believing it's the only viable option. Even though the manufacturers of Premarin and Prempro tried to hold on to the multibillion-dollar synthetic HRT market by recommending that physicians prescribe lower doses and short-term therapy with their synthetic products, millions of women began to refuse them.

Reluctantly, pharmaceutical companies brought a few natural hormones to the market in response to public demand. They even started to advertise these to physicians and to the public. In reality, their efforts to "naturalize" the pharmaceutical hormone industry were only partial. Pharmaceutically manufactured "combination natural hormone" products mix natural hormones (usually estradiol) with a synthetic progestin in order to fulfill the requirements for patent protection. Eventually, however, a number of such combo natural–synthetic products proved ineffective and left the market as fallout from the Women's Health Initiative continued.

THE NATURAL HORMONE SOLUTION

Even as the Women's Health Initiative study dragged on, data published in reputable medical journals consistently questioned the safety and efficacy of Premarin and Prempro. Still, no study has been considered or conducted to look at other types of treatments—even though statistics and polls demonstrate that public demand is rapidly growing while information and research are desperately falling behind.

One of the options overlooked was natural, bioidentical hormones, with their remarkable track record of success, endorsed by highly respected and experienced physicians such as the guru of menopause Christiane Northrup, M.D., author of the best-sellers *The Wisdom of Menopause* and *Women's Bodies, Women's Wisdom*.

A survey by the North American Menopause Society in early 2002 revealed that 90 percent of women interviewed had heard about natural hormones, 71 percent believed them to be safer and with fewer side effects than their synthetic counterparts, and 62 percent even considered them to be more efficacious than synthetic hormones.

So why has our government turned a blind eye to the evaluation and study of natural hormones? In 1997, a survey conducted by Dr. Maryanne Legato from Columbia University Women's Health Center identified priorities of aging women. It clearly determined that more women deemed their top priority as they age to be better health than other areas of life they wanted to improve.

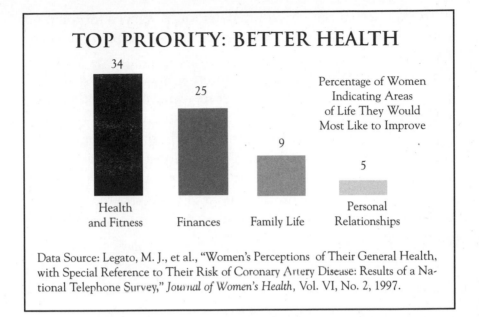

TOP PRIORITY: BETTER HEALTH

Percentage of Women
Indicating Areas
of Life They Would
Most Like to Improve

Health and Fitness: 34
Finances: 25
Family Life: 9
Personal Relationships: 5

Data Source: Legato, M. J., et al., "Women's Perceptions of Their General Health, with Special Reference to Their Risk of Coronary Artery Disease: Results of a National Telephone Survey," *Journal of Women's Health*, Vol. VI, No. 2, 1997.

With this critical information in mind, it becomes even more surprising the NIH invested so much time and resources into the WHI study without also looking at lifestyle, diet, and exercise. Keep in mind that in 1997 when this survey was conducted, exercise was becoming a national pastime and diet was rising to top priority. And still the Women's Health Initiative continued studying synthetic hormone replacement therapy alone.

By September 2002, less than three months after the announcement that the NIH was pulling the plug on the study, Premarin and Prempro seemed to go out of favor. As a result, approximately seven million women and their physicians were left in the lurch. What are the options now? Where do we go from here? And above all, whom do we trust? Even today, women's health has a long way to go, and treatment options for symptoms of hormone imbalance are not being investigated with the same interest and financial commitment there was for Prempro.

For this reason, in early August 2002, together with a group of concerned physicians, I founded the not-for-profit International Hormone Institute. Its mission is to educate women and physicians about natural hormones and create a forum of key opinion leaders in the field of women's health to determine the need for studies of various methods of treatment and research in areas of hormone imbalances.

Given the reality that forty million women are now in their perimenopausal and menopausal years—and much of their lives will be lived long after hormones have left their bodies—we must look at solutions. While the debate over hormones continues to rage, what do we do? What are our options? Is there anything women can do to prevent chronic disease, to end the symptoms of menopause, or to delay the debility of old age? Or are we doomed to just curl up and wait for the end even if it takes another forty years? I say *no!*

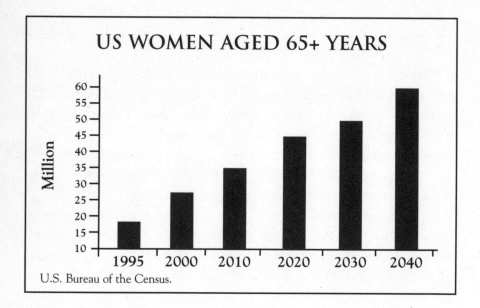

U.S. Bureau of the Census.

The U.S. Bureau of the Census publishes a yearly update on our population. By the year 2040, there will be sixty million women over sixty-five. We can no longer ignore the magnitude of their numbers or their impact on our society.

We must develop a unified approach of government-sponsored, unbiased research, looking at options and offering education and useful information. We have to eliminate partisan special-interest involvement in women's health. Full disclosure and investigation of all options must become a priority.

In the meantime, women must continue to take responsibility for their own health and welfare. If your doctor recommends that you take synthetic hormones, don't just take his or her word for it. Do your own research, and consult other doctors to get their opinions. If you were taking synthetic HRT to relieve uncomfortable symptoms of menopause, you now know that you have natural alternatives. Whichever option you choose, I urge you to work with your doctor, armed with strength and knowledge, to find the solution that works best for you.

19

A FINAL WORD

Congratulations! You've just completed the first thirty days of the program. By now, you're probably feeling stronger and more energetic; your thinking is clearer, and your outlook is brighter. You have helped eliminate many of the toxins that were building up inside you and poisoning your body while irreparably throwing your hormones out of balance. You've added a reasonable amount of exercise into your daily routine, which increased your metabolic rate. You're taking your hormones and supplements that are the fuel and substrates you need to create energy and to bolster the hormone balance you desperately need to stay young and feel good. You're writing in your journal every day, staying mindful of the changes you've made for a healthier lifestyle. You've covered all your bases.

So now you're set for the rest of your life, right? Yes and no. You know the principles you need to follow. You have the best intentions about living right. But like most people, you probably feel that unless you do everything the way it's supposed to be done, you might as well give up. One slip, and it's back to old habits. It's all or nothing, black or white.

The truth is, nothing is black or white. Life is about many shades of gray. The whole point is to enjoy life today, while you're thinking about tomorrow. Keep in mind that what you're doing today will unequivocally affect tomorrow. At the same time, you have to acknowledge that you're human. You're going to follow the plan sometimes, and go off it at other times. But if you understand the basic principles of what makes you well and what makes you ill, know how the interactions among all the factors affect you, and are watching your body and your body's reactions, you're no longer going to want to do things that are potentially destructive to your body. The point is that you want to stay alive and feel good, and that involves a new sense of awareness and responsibility. You're doing the best you can in a natural, realistic way to stay healthy while acknowledging that you live in an increasingly stressful world. Remember the concept of reasonable expectations.

If there should come a time when things aren't going so well, when adversity strikes, when stressful situations become overwhelming and you find yourself veering off course, don't despair. Go back to Week 1 of the plan. Start simply and build yourself back up to Day 30 again. Be kind to yourself. It's never too late to start again.

Glossary

Adrenal glands Two endocrine glands (see *endocrine*); they're located on top of each kidney. The inner layer (medulla) releases the hormones adrenaline (epinephrine) and norepinephrine. These hormones are released into the bloodstream during times of stress. The outer layer (cortex) produces and releases the hormones cortisol and aldosterone, and the sex hormones estrogen, progesterone, and testosterone.

Adrenaline Another term for epinephrine (see *epinephrine*).

Aldosterone A hormone produced and released by the adrenal glands. It acts on the kidneys to regulate salt and water balance. Aldosterone helps control blood pressure, the distribution of fluids in the body, and the balance of electrolytes.

Alzheimer's disease A progressive form of dementia. It is associated with diffuse degeneration of the brain over time.

Amino acids The basic building blocks of proteins. The breakdown of proteins in the human body yields amino acids. The body makes and utilizes different combinations of amino acids to build proteins of various sizes and functions. Some amino acids are made in the body; others, called essential amino acids, can only be obtained from foods high in protein.

Anabolism The synthesis or "building" of complex molecules such as proteins, fats, and carbohydrates from simpler "building blocks" like amino acids, fatty acids, and simple sugars (glucose). This process consumes and generates energy (ATP).

Androgen A type of sex hormones present in males and females. Androgens stimulate the development of sex organs and produce masculinizing characteristics (facial hair, deepening of the voice, and increased muscular development). They are secreted in small amounts by the adrenal glands (cortex) and ovaries. In fatty tissues, they are converted into estrogen. In women, excessive amounts produce masculine features such as facial hair and deep voice.

ATP (adenosine triphosphate) A "high-energy" molecule made and used by all cells in the body. ATP is formed from adenosine diphosphate (ADP) and adenosine monophosphate (AMP). ATP is the final high-energy molecule produced from the breakdown of carbohydrates or other food substances (see *catabolism*).

Bioidentical A term used to compare two compounds that are biologically equivalent in form and function. Bioidentical hormones are physiologically and chemically identical to human hormones. The molecules that make up bioidentical hormones are identical to the human hormone molecules. Bioidentical hormones are usually derived from plant sources.

Birth control (contraception) Pregnancy prevention. Birth control methods work by either preventing the ovaries from releasing the egg (ovum), preventing the implantation of the fertilized egg into the uterus, or preventing the sperm from reaching and fertilizing the ovum.

Birth control pills (oral contraceptives) A pill taken by mouth on a daily basis made of synthetic hormone molecules devised to override the body's regular cycle, preventing ovulation and pregnancy. Birth control pills do not prevent sexually transmitted diseases.

Calcitonin A hormone that helps regulate calcium metabolism. It lowers levels of calcium and phosphate in the blood by decreasing bone breakdown. Calcitonin is produced by and released from the thyroid gland.

Calcium An element found in nature and used by the body to form bones and teeth. Calcium is directly involved in many metabolic processes, including fat metabolism, nerve transmission, skeletal muscle contraction (tightening), proper heart function, and blood clot formation. A lack of calcium may lead to brittle and weak bones (see *osteoporosis*), irregular heartbeats (arrhythmia), or prolonged bleeding.

Calendar method A method of birth control that estimates ovulation based on previous menstrual cycles. This information is used to predict which days of the month a woman is most fertile, typically twenty-four to forty-eight hours after ovulation.

Carbohydrates A large group of compounds that include sugars and starches. All carbohydrates are broken down in the body from complex structures to basic building blocks (glucose). Simple carbohydrates are sugars that are naturally found in fruits (fructose), vegetables (sucrose), and dairy (lactose). They are also found in breads, cereals, sauces, candies, and pastries. Complex carbohydrates are primarily starches, some of which include flour, whole-grain breads, rice, pasta, potatoes, beans, and fruits and vegetables. Carbohydrates are essential to all cellular processes in the body.

Catabolism A process involving chemical breakdown of complex substances to form simpler ones, involving significant use of energy (ATP). The substances broken down include foods (carbohydrates, protein, fats, and so forth) as well as the body's own storage products (glycogen, fats, and more).

Cervical cap A contraceptive made of rubber and shaped like a large thimble. It fits tightly over the cervix. It is used with a spermicidal gel or cream and prevents the sperm from reaching the uterus and thus the egg. Cervical caps do not prevent sexually transmitted diseases.

Cholesterol The precursor of steroid hormones such as glucocorticoids, mineralocorticoids, and sex hormones.

Compound A substance made of two or more parts, ingredients, or materials.

Compounding A pharmaceutical process by which a custom preparation is made following a doctor's prescription. These formulations are not mass-produced (precompounded) by large pharmaceutical companies.

Conjugated equine estrogens A mixture of specific metabolic waste products of estrogens that are extracted from the urine of pregnant horses; Premarin is one example.

Constipation A condition in which the evacuation of the bowel occurs infrequently. Bowel movements vary from person to person. Constipation is considered to occur when normal bowel habits of an individual become infrequent, painful, or difficult.

Corticosteroid Any steroid hormone synthesized by the adrenal gland (cortex). The glucocorticoids (hydrocortisone, cortisol, cortisone, corticosterone) are essential for the utilization of carbohydrates, fats, and proteins for a normal response to stress. The mineralocorticoids (aldosterone) are necessary for the regulation of salt and water balance. See *cholesterol*.

Cortisol See *corticosteroid*.

Designer hormones Synthetic hormone compounds manufactured by pharmaceutical companies designed to target specific organs with specific hormone actions.

DHEA (dihydro-epiandrosterone) A hormone precursor of testosterone.

Diabetes A common disorder of carbohydrate metabolism that is caused by inadequate insulin quality and/or quantity. As a result, the level of sugar (glucose) in the blood is too high (hyperglycemia) (see *insulin*). Type 2 diabetes (also called adult-onset diabetes or non-insulin-dependent diabetes mellitus—NIDDM) is usually associated with obesity, sedentary lifestyle, and poor dietary habits. In contrast, type 1 diabetes (also called juvenile-onset diabetes—IDDM) is a disorder cause by a deficiency of insulin production and insulin resistance.

Diaphragm (mechanical contraception) A dome-shaped device made of rubber with a firm, flexible rim. It fits inside a woman's vagina and covers the cervix. It is used in combination with a sperm-killing (spermicidal) cream or jelly. It does not protect against sexually transmitted diseases.

Diet The type and combination of foods a person eats. A balanced diet contains adequate quantities of all nutrients. A *diet* may also be used to describe behavior and actions associated with the consumption of food—for instance, "He is on a diet."

Dietary supplement A vitamin or other substance naturally occurring in the human body that is added to the diet in either pill, powder, or liquid form. Supplements are not necessarily used to treat specific dietary deficiencies. Unlike prescription medications, dietary supplements are not controlled by the Food and Drug Administration.

Dopamine A hormone produced during the synthesis of norepinephrine. It appears in adrenal glands and in the brain.

Efficacy The effect of a drug, vitamin, or supplement vis-à-vis the expected reaction.

Electrolytes Elements found in the body. They include potassium, calcium, sodium, and magnesium. Electrolytes must exist in fixed balance to maintain the body's fluid balance, heart rhythm, muscle activity, and all metabolic function.

Endocrine gland (ductless gland) A gland that manufactures one or more hormones and secretes them directly into the bloodstream. The thyroid, adrenals, ovaries, testes, pituitary, and part of the pancreas are considered endocrine glands.

Endocrinology The study of endocrine glands, hormones, and diseases caused by excessive or deficient amounts of hormones.

Endometrium The lining of the uterus. It progressively becomes thicker and more glandular with an increased blood supply in the second half of the menstrual cycle.

Enzyme A protein whose function is to mediate and enhance specific chemical reactions in the body.

Epinephrine (adrenaline) A hormone secreted by the adrenal gland. Its effect is to increase metabolism, heart rate, blood pressure, and blood flow to large muscles. Epinephrine release helps with the "fight or flight" response to stress.

Estradiol (E_2) The most active and dominant type of estrogen produced in the ovaries. It is produced in large quantities by young women.

Estriol (E_3) A relatively weak estrogen. It is the dominant hormone of pregnancy.

Estrogen(s) A group of hormones with feminizing effects in the body (breast development, cellular growth, ovulation, fertilization, fat deposition, and so on).

Estrone (E_1) The estrogen hormone that's produced around menopause. It's largely available from the conversion of androgens in fatty tissues.

Fatigue A feeling of tiredness, exhaustion, and lack of energy.

Fatty acids The building blocks of fats. Like amino acids, most fatty acids are synthesized in the body. Essential fatty acids must be obtained from the diet; they cannot be made in the body.

Fertility A woman's ability to become pregnant.

Fiber Dietary fiber consists of indigestible carbohydrates such as cellulose, derived primarily from plants. It adds bulk to food and draws fluid into the digestive tract, both of which help with bowel movement regularity. Fiber also interferes with fat absorption and prevents rapid sugar-level rise in the bloodstream by delaying sugar absorption.

Fibroids Benign growths in the muscular lining or cavity of the uterus.

Follicle The area in the ovary where the egg (ovum) matures and prepares for ovulation.

Follicle-stimulating hormone (FSH) A hormone that stimulates the development of the egg while in the ovary. It also directly affects estrogen production in the ovaries. In men, FSH helps control the production of sperm.

Follicular phase or early phase of the menstrual cycle. It follows menstruation while the egg matures. It is characterized by a slow rise in estrogen levels.

Gastrin A hormone produced by special cells (G cells) in the lining of the stomach. Gastrin levels rise when food enters the stomach and triggers the release of stomach acid (gastric acid). Stomach acid (hydrochloric) helps break down food for digestion.

Glucagon A hormone produced by the pancreas that causes the liver to release its stored sugar (glycogen) into the bloodstream during times of low sugar levels (hypoglycemia) or starvation.

Gluten A protein found in grains such as wheat, barley, and rye.

Gonadotropin-releasing hormone (GnRH) A hormone released from the hypothalamus into the pituitary circulation. GnRH prompts the release of both follicle-stimulating hormone (FSH) and luteinizing hormone (LH).

Gonadotropins (gonadotropic hormones) Any sex hormones that have been released by the pituitary gland to stimulate the sex organs (ovaries or testes) to release the hormones they manufacture (estrogen, progesterone, and testosterone).

Gonads Reproductive glands (ovaries and testes).

Growth hormone (GH) A hormone produced by the pituitary gland essential for growth and metabolism. GH levels drop with age.

Homeostasis The physiological process by which the body maintains internal equilibrium.

Hormone Substance produced by cells that circulates in the bloodstream and body fluids and exerts specific effects on cells elsewhere in the body. Hormones are our bodies' messengers. They tell our organs, cells, and tissues what to do and when to do it.

Hormone replacement therapy (HRT) The replacement by an outside source of one or more hormones depleted in the body. The term is used to refer to treatment with synthetic hormones.

Hot flash A sudden feeling of heat caused by the rapid dilation of capillaries under the skin and associated with sudden fluctuations in hormone levels.

Hysterectomy The surgical procedure by which the uterus only is removed.

Immune system The body's natural defense system. When working properly, the immune system allows the body to successfully fight off infections of bacterial or viral origin.

Inertia Sluggishness or absence of activity.

Insomnia The inability to fall asleep or remain asleep for an adequate length of time.

Insulin A hormone that helps regulate sugar (glucose) levels in the body. It is released when the level of sugar (glucose) in the blood rises. High insulin levels correlate to low blood sugar levels.

Intrauterine device (IUD) A small plastic and metal device that is inserted inside the uterus. A nylon string at the end of the IUD passes through the opening of the uterus (the cervix) into the vagina. IUDs mechanically prevent implantation of the egg into the uterus. Some IUDs contain synthetic hormones.

L-carnitine A naturally occurring amino acid required in energy production. L-carnitine transports fatty acids inside the cell to the cellular energy factories (mitochondria), where they are used for energy production. L-carnitine is also important in the production of all hormones.

Libido Level of sexual interest in men and women.

Luteinizing hormone (LH) A hormone produced by the pituitary gland that stimulates ovulation as well as the production of progesterone by the ovaries and testosterone by the testes.

Magnesium An electrolyte—an element essential to life—magnesium is involved in chemical reactions directly responsible for effective functioning of muscles, nerves, brain, heart, and overall metabolism.

Mammography A low-radiation-dose X ray of the breasts designed to uncover abnormalities.

Medroxyprogesterone A synthetic female sex hormone (progestin). It is used as part of synthetic hormone replacement therapy.

Melatonin A hormone produced by a small gland (pineal) in the brain. It participates in the regulation of sleep-wake cycles.

Menarche The age at onset of menstruation.

Menopause The normal cessation of the menstrual cycle in women, occurring usually in the late forties and early fifties. Clinically, it's defined as the time after a woman has not had a period for a year. Any correlation between the presence or absence of menstruation and symptoms of hormone imbalance is minimal.

Menstrual cycle Usually twenty-eight to thirty days in length; the term refers to the changes that take place in a women's body between two menstrual periods.

Metabolism The sum of all the physical and chemical processes occurring in the body: anabolism and catabolism.

Micronize A term derived from the Greek word *micron*, a small thing. In pharmaceuticals, it refers to small particle sizes. Micronized progesterone and testosterone are bioidentical/natural hormones in minute particle size.

Neurotransmitters Chemicals that provide communication among nerve cells within the nervous system.

Oil of evening primrose Oil derived from the *Oenothera biennis* plant. It may help relieve premenstrual syndrome symptoms (PMS), including breast discomfort. The oil of evening primrose is a rich source of gamma-linolenic acid (GLA), an essential fatty acid.

Omega-3 fatty acids Fatty acids found in marine plant and fish. EPA (eicosapentaenoic acid) and DHA (docosahexenoic acid) are examples of omega-3 fatty acids and are ingredients in fish oil supplements. They may improve cell membrane integrity and neuro-transmission; mood; and hair and nail integrity.

Oophorectomy (ovariectomy) Surgical removal of an ovary or ovaries.

Osteopenia A low bone mass.

Osteoporosis A loss of bony tissue, resulting in bones that are brittle and thin. Generalized osteoporosis is common in elderly people with poor diets and on multiple medications, including steroids. Loss of hormones during menopause may be associated with potential increased risk of osteoporosis.

Ovaries The pair of female reproductive organs on both sides of the pelvis that produce eggs and secrete sex hormones.

Ovulation The release of an egg from the ovarian follicle fourteen days before the beginning of menstruation: the point in time in which fertilization can occur.

Parathyroid glands Two pairs of endocrine glands below or in the thyroid gland. The parathyroid glands produce a hormone called parathyroid hormone or PTH.

Parathyroid hormone A hormone produced by the parathyroid gland. It helps regulate calcium and phosphorus levels in the blood. It directly affects bone health.

Perimenopause A term used to describe the period of time just before menopause; it may last as long as several years.

Pharmacist A person practicing the profession of pharmacy. It includes the preparation, compounding, and dispensing of drugs.

Phytohormones Hormones derived from plants. *Phyto* is derived from the Greek word for "plant."

Pituitary gland The endocrine gland located in the brain that produces thyroid-stimulating hormone (TSH), adrenocorticotrophic hormone (ACTH), growth hormone (GH), gonadotropins (FSH, LH), and prolactin. See *thyroid-stimulating hormone*.

Placebo An inert substance used instead of an active ingredient in studies of medication effects.

Polycystic ovary syndrome A medical condition defined as multiple cysts in the ovaries, irregular menstruation, insulin resistance, fertility issues, and multiple symptoms of hormone imbalance.

Progesterone A hormone produced by the ovaries during and after ovulation. Progesterone helps prepare the lining of the uterus to receive a fertilized egg. If the egg does not get fertilized, progesterone levels drop and menstruation starts. Progesterone is the balance for estrogen effects—it's used to balance the effects of estrogen in a hormone supplementation regime.

Progestin A synthetic version of progesterone possessing minimal similarity to the molecular structure of progesterone. It's used in synthetic hormone replacement therapy.

Prostate-specific antigen (PSA) A cellular receptor substance. A measurement of prostate gland cell growth and cellular turnover.

Protein One of the main food ingredients, made up of amino acids. Proteins are critical to the manufacture of cells, production of energy, building of muscles and hormones, support of the immune system, and maintenance of bone structure as well as heart and brain function.

Receptor A specific area on the surface of a cell that provides a specific fit to certain proteins, hormones, enzymes, or other substances important to the cellular function.

Renin A hormone produced by the kidney that helps increase blood pressure.

Rhythm method A contraceptive method in which sexual intercourse is restricted to the safe period, typically the beginning and end of menstruation. Measurement of basal body temperature is used to help determine time of ovulation; this temperature rises suddenly when ovulation has occurred. The fertile period is the following twenty-four to forty-eight hours.

Steroid A substance whose chemical formula is similar to cortisol. Pharmaceutical derivatives such as prednisone and anabolic steroids are synthetically manufactured.

Systemic Related to or affecting the body as a whole.

Testosterone A sex hormone present in both men and women, but dominant in men. Produced in the testes and adrenal glands, it's directly responsible for sperm production, muscle development, facial hair and body hair, and male personality traits. The ovaries in women produce testosterone in smaller amounts.

Thyroid-stimulating hormone (TSH) A pituitary hormone that stimulates the production of thyroid hormones by the thyroid gland.

Uterus (womb) The part of the female reproductive tract that allows the fertilized egg to become implanted in its wall (endometrium). After successful implantation, the uterus supports the fertilized egg while it matures into a fetus and is delivered as a newborn baby after a forty-week gestation period.

Vaginal atrophy As a result of loss of proper hormone balance, the vaginal walls become thin and dry. Topical treatment may not relieve the problem; systemic hormone supplementation offers a better option.

Vitamins Organic compounds that help perform specific metabolic functions. The body cannot make vitamins, so they are obtained from the diet or from supplementation.

Resources

ERIKA SCHWARTZ M.D.

www.drerika.com

NATURAL HORMONES

www.naturalhormonepharmacy.com
www.hormonesolution.com
www.nhpinfo.com

For more information regarding Long Island cancer research, visit the National Cancer Institute:
http://epi.grants.cancer.gov/LIBCSP
www.nci.nih.gov/cancerinfo/LIBCSP

ONLINE COMMUNITIES FOR WOMEN

The Power-Surge Community for Women at Midlife and Menopause
http://www.power-surge.com

Christiane Northrup, M.D.
http://www.drnorthrup.com

SKIN CARE

Skinklinic
8006 Fifth Avenue
New York, NY 10021
(212) 521-3100

ORGANIZATIONS

North American Menopause Society
www.menopause.org
P.O. Box 94527
Cleveland, OH 44101
(440) 442-7550
fax (440) 442-2660

American Menopause Foundation
http://www.americanmenopause.org
350 Fifth Avenue, Suite 2822
New York, NY 10018
(212) 714-2398
fax (212) 714-1252

National Women's Health Network
www.womenshealthnetwork.org
514 10th Street NW
Suite 400 (4th Floor)
Washington, DC 20004
(202) 347-1140
fax (202) 347-1168

For international menopause web references, visit:
www.womanlab.com

International Hormone Institute
www.drerika.com

COMPOUNDING PHARMACIES

The Natural Hormone Pharmacy
200 Saw Mill River Road
Hawthorne, NY 10532
(800) 522-6692
www.naturalhormonepharmacy.com

For OTC product lines, contact:
Dr. Erika's Essential Elements
www.drerika.com
(914) 747-1842

Ecological Formulas
(800) 351-9429

Life Extension Foundation
(800) 544-4440

Metagenics
www.metagenics.com
(800) 638-2848

Symbiotics, Inc.
www.symbiotics.com
(928) 203-0277

Recommended Reading

Michael Blumenfield, M.D., and Maria L.A. Tiamson M.D., *Consultation-Liaison Psychiatry* (Practical Guides in Psychiatry series). Lippincott, Williams & Wilkins, 2003.

Jonny Bowden, *Shape Up! The 8-Week Plan to Transform Your Body, Your Health and Your Life*. Perseus Publishing, 2001.

Ellen Brown and Lynn Walker, *Menopause and Estrogen: Natural Alternatives to Hormone Replacement Therapy*. Frog, Ltd., 1996.

Robert N. Butler, M.D., and Myrna Lewis, *The New Love and Sex After 60*. Ballantine Books, 2002.

Laura E. Corio and Linda G. Kahn, *The Change Before the Change: Everything You Need to Know to Stay Healthy in the Decade Before Menopause*. Bantam Doubleday Dell, 2000.

R. Cotrell, *Stress Management* (Wellness series). McGraw-Hill/Dushkin, 1992.

Ellie Cullen, *Normal Blood Test Scores Aren't Good Enough*. YFH Press, 2002.

S. Boyd Eaton, Marjorie Shostak, and Melvin J. Konner, *The Paleolithic Prescription*. HarperCollins, 1988.

The Editors of Prevention Magazine Health Books, *New Choices in Natural Healing: Over 1,800 of the Best Self-Help Remedies from the World of Alternative Medicine*. Rodale Press, 1997.

Oz Garcia and Sharyn Kolberg, *Look and Feel Fabulous Forever: The World's Best Supplements, Anti-Aging Techniques, and High-Tech Health Secrets*. ReganBooks, 2001.

Oz Garcia and Sharyn Kolberg, *The Balance: Your Personal Prescription for Supermetabolism, Renewed Vitality, Maximum Health, Instant Rejuvenation*. ReganBooks, 1998.

James Jamieson, *Growth Hormone: The Methuselah Factor*. Safe Goods, 1998.

B. Kliman, R. Vermette, and E. Kolowrat, *What You Should Know About Medical Lab Tests*. T. Y. Crowell, 1979.

Miriam E. Nelson, *Strong Women Stay Young*. Bantam Doubleday Dell, 2000.

Christiane Northrup, M.D., *The Wisdom of Menopause: Creating Physical and Emotional Health and Healing During the Change*. Bantam Doubleday Dell, 2001.

Christiane Northrup, M.D., *Women's Bodies, Women's Wisdom: Creating Physical and Emotional Health and Healing*. Bantam Books, 1998 (rev. ed.).

Rosemarie Schulman and Harold Schulman, *Tipping the Scales: Getting Answers on Weight Management*. Xlibris Corporation, 2002.

Erika Schwartz, M.D., *The Hormone Solution: Naturally Alleviate Symptoms of Hormone Imbalance from Adolescence through Menopause*. Warner Books, 2002.

Erika Schwartz, M.D., and Carol Colman, *Natural Energy: From Tired to Terrific in 10 Days*. Putnam, 1999.

Bernie S. Siegel, M.D., *Love, Medicine & Miracles: Lessons Learned about Self-Healing from a Surgeon's Experience with Exceptional Patients*. HarperCollins, 1986.

Andrew Weil, M.D., *Eating Well for Optimum Health: The Essential Guide to Bringing Health and Pleasure Back to Eating*. Quill, 2001.

References

PREFACE

Schwartz, Erika. *The Hormone Solution: Naturally Alleviate Symptoms of Hormone Imbalance from Adolescence through Menopause.* Warner Books, 2002.

Writing Group for the Women's Health Initiative Investigators. "Risks and benefits of estrogen plus progestin in healthy postmenopausal women: Principal results from the Women's Health Initiative randomized controlled trial." *Journal of the American Medical Association* July 17, 2002; 28:3:321–333.

CHAPTER 1: WHAT EVERYONE NEEDS TO KNOW

Krimsky, Sheldon. *Hormonal Chaos: The Scientific and Social Origins of the Environmental Endocrine Hypothesis.* Johns Hopkins University Press, 1999.

Berkson, Lindsey D., and John A. McLachlan. *Hormone Deception: How Everyday Foods and Products Are Disrupting Your Hormones—How to Protect Yourself and Your Family.* Contemporary Books, 2001.

Endocrine Disruptors Research Initiative. http://www.epa.gov/ endocrine.

Garcia, Oz, and Sharyn Kolberg. *Look and Feel Fabulous Forever: The World's Best Supplements, Anti-Aging Techniques, and High-Tech Health Secrets*. ReganBooks, 2001.

Schwartz, Erika, and Carol Colman. *Natural Energy: From Tired to Terrific in 10 Days*. Putnam, 1999.

Wilson, Robert. *Feminine Forever*. M. Evans & Company, 1968.

Lee, John R., Virginia Hopkins, and Jesse Hanley. *What Your Doctor May Not Tell You About Premenopause*. Warner Books, 1999.

Corio, Laura E., and Linda G. Kahn. *The Change Before The Change: Everything You Need to Know to Stay Healthy in the Decade Before Menopause*. Bantam Doubleday Dell, 2000.

Northrup, Christiane. *The Wisom of Menopause: Creating Physical and Emotional Health and Healing During the Change*. Bantam Doubleday Dell, 2001.

Northrup, Christiane. *Women's Bodies,Women's Wisdom: Creating Physical and Emotional Health and Healing*. Bantam Books, 1998.

Schwartz, Erika. *The Hormone Solution: Naturally Alleviate Symptoms of Hormone Imbalance from Adolescence through Menopause*. Warner Books, 2002.

Cullen, Ellie. *Normal Blood Test Scores Aren't Good Enough*. YFH Press, 2002.

Chase, M., et al., "Blood work reveals just how healthy or sick you are." *Wall Street Journal Health Journal* Jan. 22, 1996.

Kliman, B., R. Vermette, and E. Kolowrat. *What You Should Know About Medical Lab Tests*. T.Y. Crowell, 1979.

CHAPTER 2: HOW YOUR LIFE AFFECTS YOUR HORMONES

Henry, J.P. "Biological basis of the stress response." *Integrated Physiological Behavioral Sciences* 1992; 27:1:66–83.

Krimsky, Sheldon. *Hormonal Chaos: The Scientific and Social Origins of the Environmental Endocrine Hypothesis*. Johns Hopkins University Press, 1999.

Berkson, Lindsey D., and John A. McLachlan. *Hormone Deception: How Everyday Foods and Products Are Disrupting Your Hormones—and How to Protect Yourself and Your Family*. Contemporary Books, 2001.

Endocrine Disruptors Research Initiative. http://www.epa.gov/endocrine.

Long Island Breast Cancer Study Project. http://www.epi.grants.cancer.gov/LIBCSP.

Willet, W.C., Rochhill. B., Hankinson, S.E., et al. "Epidemiology and nongenetic causes of breast cancer." In *Diseases of the Breast*, Harris, J.R., Lippman, M.E., Morrow, M., and Osborne C.K. (eds.). Lippincott, Williams & Wilkins, 2000, p. 175.

Band, P., Le, N., Fang, R., and Deschamps, M. "Carcinogenic and endocrine disrupting effects of cigarette smoke and risk of breast cancer." *Lancet* 2002; 360:1044.

Collaborative Group on Hormonal Factors in Breast Cancer. "Alcohol, tobacco and breast cancer: Collaborative reanalysis of individual data from 53 epidemiological studies, including 58,515 women with breast cancer and 95,067 women without the disease." *British Journal of Cancer* 2002; 87:1234.

Ron, E., Lubin, J.H., Shore, R.E., et al. "Thyroid cancer after exposure to external radiation: A pooled analysis of seven studies." *Radiation Resident* 1995; 141:259.

Hancock, S.L., Cox, R.S., McDougall, I.R. "Thyroid diseases after treatment of Hodgkin's disease." *New England Journal of Medicine* 1991; 325:599.

Sklar, C., Whitton, J., Mertens, A., et al. "Abnormalities of the thyroid in survivors of Hodgkin's disease: Data from the Childhood Cancer Survivor Study." *Journal of Clinical Endocrinology and Metabolism* 2000; 85:3227.

Hall, P., Holm, L.E. "Late consequences of radioiodine for diagnosis and therapy in Sweden." *Thyroid* 1997; 7:205.

Robbins, J., Schneider, A.B. "Thyroid cancer following exposure to radioactive iodine." *Reviews of Endocrinological and Metabolical Diseases* 2000; 1:197.

Born, J., et al. "Effects of sleep and circadian rhythm on human circulating immune cells." *Journal of Immunology* 1997; 158: 4454–4464.

Spiegel, K., et al. "Impact of sleep debt on metabolic and endocrine function." *Lancet* Oct. 23, 1999; 354:1435–1439.

Levine, J.P. "Putting WHI into perspective: What to tell patients about HRT critical issues in menopause." *Female Patient* Dec. 2002.

CHAPTER 3: THE NATURAL HORMONE SOLUTION

Schwartz, Erika. *The Hormone Solution: Naturally Alleviate Symptoms of Hormone Imbalance from Adolescence through Menopause.* Warner Books, 2002.

Writing Group for the Women's Health Investigators. "Risks and benefits of estrogen plus progestin in healthy postmenopausal women: Principal results from the Women's Health Initiative randomized controlled trial." *Journal of the American Medical Association* July 17, 2002; 28:321–333.

Writing Group for the PEPI Trial. "Effects of estrogen or estrogen/progestin regimens on heart disease risk factors in postmenopausal women: The Postmenopausal Estrogen/Progestin Intervention (PEPI) Trial." *Journal of the American Medical Association* Jan. 18, 1995; 273:3:199–208.

Levine J.P. "Putting WHI into perspective: What to tell patients about HRT critical issues in menopause." *Female Patient* Dec. 2002.

Miller, P., Boling, E.P., Canalis, E., Lambing, C.L., Nichols, K.J., Schiff, I. "HRT: Not so heartily recommended." *Harvard Health Letter* Dec. 2002; 28:2:6.

Hamdy, R., et al. "Women's Health Initiative Study." *Southern Medical Journal* 2002; 95:5:951–965.

Greendale, G.A., Reboussin, B.A., Hogan, P., et al. "Symptom relief and side effects of postmenopausal hormones: Results from the Postmenopausal Estrogen/Progestin Interventions Trial." *Obstetrics and Gynecology* 1998; 92:6:982–988.

Krimsky, Sheldon. *Hormonal Chaos: The Scientific and Social Origins of the Environmental Endocrine Hypothesis.* Johns Hopkins University Press, 1999.

Hargrove, J.T., et al. "Menopausal hormone replacement therapy with continuous daily oral micronized estradiol and progesterone." *Obstetrics and Gynecology* 1989; 73:4.

CHAPTER 5: FEEDING YOUR HORMONES

Critser, Greg. *Fat Land: How Americans Became the Fattest People in the World.* Houghton Mifflin Company, 2003.

Beck, M.J., Evans, B.J., Quarry-Horn, J.L., et al. "Type 2 diabetes mellitus: Issues for the medical care of pediatric and adult patients." *Southern Medical Journal* 2002; 95:9:992–1000.

Lemonick, M.D. "Teens before their time." *Time Magazine* Oct. 30, 2000.

"Girls' body fat at age 5 linked to earlier puberty." *Reuters Health* April 8, 2003.

Krahnstoever, K.D., Susman, E.J., Lipps, L.B. "Percent body fat at age 5 predicts earlier pubertal development among girls at age 9." *Pediatrics* 2003; 111:815–821.

Atkins, Robert. *Dr. Atkins' New Diet Revolution.* Avon, 2001 (revised edition).

Ornish, D., et al. "Low-fat diets." *New England Journal of Medicine* Jan. 8, 1998; 338:127–129.

Jeppesen, J., et al. "Effects of low-fat, high-carbohydrate diets on risk factors for ischemic heart disease in postmenopausal women." *American Journal of Clinical Nutrition* 1997; 65:1027–1033.

Schwartz, Erika, and Carol Colman. *Natural Energy: From Tired to Terrific in 10 Days*. Putnam, 1998.

Katan, M.B., et al. "Beyond low-fat diets." *New England Journal of Medicine* Aug. 21, 1997; 337:563–566.

Morgan, S.A., et al. "A low-fat diet supplemented with monosaturated fat results in less HDL-C lowering than a very-low-fat diet." *Journal of the American Dietetic Association* 1997; 97:2:151–156.

Von Schacky, C., Angerer, P., Kothny, W, et al. "The effect of dietary omega-3 fatty acids on coronary atherosclerosis: A randomized, double-blind, placebo-controlled trial." *Annals of Internal Medicine* 1999; 130:554–562.

Nair, S.D., Leitch, J.W., Falconer, J., et al. "Prevention of cardiac arrhythmia by dietary (N-3) polyunsaturated fatty acids and their mechanism of action." *Journal of Nutrition* 1997; 127:383–393.

Leaf, A., Weber, P.C., et al. "Cardiovascular effects of N-3 fatty acids." *New England Journal of Medicine* 1988; 318:549–557.

Nelson, G.J., et al. "Low-fat diets do not lower plasma cholesterol levels in healthy men compared to high-fat diets with similar fatty acid composition at constant caloric intake." *Lipids* 1995; 30:11:969–976.

Nettleton, J.A., et al. "Omega 3 fatty acids: Comparison of plant and seafood sources in human nutrition." *Journal of the American Dietetic Association* 1991; 91:331–333.

Rimm, E.B., et al. "Vegetable, fruit, and cereal fiber intake and risk of coronary heart disease among men." *Journal of the American Medical Association* 1996; 275:6:447–451.

CHAPTER 6: EXERCISE

Stahl, S.M. "Sex and psychopharmacology: Is natural estrogen a psychotropic drug in women?" *Archives of General Psychiatry* 2001; 58:537–538.

Maes, M., Smith, R., Christophe, A., et al. "Fatty acid composition in major depression: Decreased omega 3 fractions in cholesteryl esters and increased C20:4 Omega 6/C20:5 omega 3 ratio in cholesteryl esters and phospholipids." *Journal of Affective Disorders* 1996; 38:35–46.

Marano, H.E. "Depression: Beyond serotonin." *Psychology Today* March–April 1999; 30–76.

CHAPTER 7: SUPPLEMENTS

Schwartz, Erika, and Carol Colman. *Natural Energy: From Tired to Terrific in 10 Days*. Putnam, 1998.

Ferrari, R., S. DiMauro, and G. Sherwood, eds. *L-Carnitine and Its Role in Medicine: From Function to Therapy*. Academic Press, 1992.

"Fish oil may help relieve depression." *Internal Medicine World Report* Dec. 2002; A:12:31.

Chevaux, K.A., Song, W.O. "Adrenocortical function and cholesterol in pantothenic acid deficiency." *Federation of American Societies for Experimental Biology* 1994; 8:2588.

Snider, B.L., Dieteman, D.F. "Pyridoxide therapy for premenstrual acne flare." *Archive of Dermatology* 1974; 110:130–131.

Eaton, S. Boyd, Marjorie Shostak, and Melvin J. Konner. *The Paleolithic Prescription*. HarperCollins, 1988.

Okuda, K., Yashima, K., Kitazaki, T., et al. "Intestinal absorption and concurrent chemical changes of methylcobalamin." *Journal of Laboratory Clinical Medicine* 1973; 81:557–567.

Heaney, R., Recker, R. "Distribution of calcium absorption in middle-aged women." *American Journal of Clinical Nutrition* 1986; 43:299–305.

Curhan, G.C., Willett, W.C., Rimm, E.B., et al. "A prospective study of dietary calcium and other nutrients and the risks of symptomatic kidney stones." *New England Journal of Medicine* 1993; 328:880–882.

Lloyd, T., Andon, M.B., Rollis, N., et al. "Calcium supplementation and bone mineral density in adolescent girls." *Journal of the American Medical Association* 1993; 270:841–844.

Durlach, J., Durlach, V., Bac, P., et al. "Magnesium and therapeutics." *Magnesium Research* 1994; 7:313–328.

Dyckner, T., Wester, P.O., et al. "Effect of magnesium on blood pressure." *British Medicine* 1983; 286:1847–1849.

Cohen, L., Laor, L., Kitzes, R., et al. "Magnesium malabsorption in postmenopausal osteoporosis." *Magnesium* 1983; 2:139–143.

Facchinetti, F., Borella, P., Sances, G., et al. "Oral magnesium successfully relieves premenstrual mood changes." *Obstetrics and Gynecology* 1991; 78:177–181.

Hambidge, M. "Human zinc deficiency." *Journal of Nutrition* 2000; 130:S1344–1349.

Sandstead, H.H. "Is zinc deficiency a public health problem?" *Nutrition* 1995; 11:87–92.

Kaplan, J., Hess, J.W., Prasad, A.S., et al. "Impairment of immune function in the elderly: Association with mild zinc deficiency." In *Essential and Toxic Trace Elements in Human Health and Disease*, Prasad, A.S. (ed.). John Wiley & Sons, 1988, pp. 309–317.

Prasad, A.S., et al. "Zinc: the biology and therapeutics of an icon." *Annals of Internal Medicine* 1996; 125:142–144.

Jamieson, James. *Growth Hormone: The Methuselah Factor*. Safe Goods, 1998.

Ferrari, R., S. DiMauro, and G. Sherwood, eds. *L-Carnitine and Its Role in Medicine: From Function to Therapy*. Academic Press, 1997.

CHAPTER 9: THE JOURNEY BEGINS: DAYS 1–5

Schwartz, Erika. *The Hormone Solution: Naturally Alleviate Symptoms of Hormone Imbalance from Adolescence through Menopause*. Warner Books, 2002.

CHAPTER 10: GETTING INTO GEAR: DAYS 6–10

Born, J., et al. "Effects of sleep and circadian rhythm on human circulating immune cells." *Journal of Immunology* 1997; 158: 4454–4464.

Moldofsky, H. "Sleep and the immune system." *International Journal of Immunopharmacology* Aug. 1995; 17:8:649–654.

Spiegel, K., et al. "Impact of sleep debt on metabolic and endocrine function." *Lancet* Oct. 23, 1999; 354:1435–1439.

Wiley, T.S., and B. Formby. *Lights Out: Sleep, Sugar, and Survival*. Pocket Books, 2000.

Von Treuer, K., et al. "Overnight human plasma melatonin, cortisol, prolactin, TSH under conditions of normal sleep, sleep deprivation, and sleep recovery." *Journal of Pineal Research* Jan. 1996; 20:1:7–14.

Montplaisir, J., Lorrain, J., Denesle, R., Petit, D. "Sleep in menopause: differential effects of two forms of hormone replacement." *Menopause* Jan. 2001; 8:1:10–16.

CHAPTER 17: AND LIFE GOES ON . . .

Spiegel, K., et al. "Impact of sleep debt on metabolic and endocrine function." *Lancet* Oct. 23, 1999; 354:1435–1439.

Von Treuer, K., et al. "Overnight human plasma melatonin, cortisol, prolactin, TSH under conditions of normal sleep, sleep deprivation, and sleep recovery." *Journal of Pineal Research* Jan. 1996; 20:1:7–14.

CHAPTER 18: SYNTHETIC SUICIDE

Woodruff, J.D., Pickar, J.H. "Incidence of endometrial hyperplasia in postmenopausal women taking conjugated estrogens (Premarin) with medroxyprogesterone acetate or conjugated estrogens alone." *American Journal of Obstetrics and Gynecology* May 1994; 170:5, Pt. 1:1213–1223.

Women's Health Initiative Study Group. "Design of the Women's Health Initiative clinical trial and observational study." *Controlled Clinical Trials* 1998; 19:61–109.

Writing Group for the Women's Health Initiative Investigators. "Risks and benefits of estrogen plus progestin in healthy postmenopausal women: Principal results from the Women's Health Initiative randomized control trial." *Journal of the American Medical Association* 2002; 28:3:321–333.

Writing Group for the PEPI Trial. "Effects of Estrogen or estrogen/progestin regimens on heart disease risk factors in postmenopausal women: The Postmenopausal Estrogen/Progestin Interventions (PEPI) Trial." *Journal of the American Medical Association* Jan. 23, 1995; 273:3:199–208.

Halpern, S.D., Karlawish, J.H.T., Berlin J. "The continuing unethical conduct of underpowered clinical trials." *Journal of the American Medical Association* 2002; 288:3:358–362.

Fletcher, S.W., Colditz, C.A. "Failure of estrogen plus progestin for prevention." *Journal of the American Medical Association* 2002; 288:3:366–368.

Lacey, J.V., Mink, P.J., Lubin, J.H., et al. "Menopausal hormone replacement therapy and risk of ovarian cancer." *Journal of the American Medical Association* 2002; 288:3:334–341.

Partridge, A.H., Winer, E.P. "Informing clinical trial participants about study results." *Journal of the American Medical Association* 2002; 288:3:358–365.

Hamdy, R., et al. "Women's Health Initiative Study." *Southern Medical Journal* 2002; 95:5:951–965.

Frieden, J., et al. "Hormone therapy study raises concerns." *Internal Medicine World Report* Dec. 2002; 26.

Levine, J.P. "Putting WHI into perspective: What to tell patients about HRT critical issues in menopause." *Female Patient* Dec. 2002.

Hendrix, S.L. "Implications of the Women's Health Initiative." *Female Patient* Nov. 2002; 4–8.

Moon, M.A. "WHI researchers defend their findings on HRT." *Clinical Rounds* Nov. 15, 2002; 14.

Rulin, M.C. "Risk of endometrial hyperplasia progressing to cancer." *American Journal of Obstetrics and Gynecology* 1995; 172:4, Pt. 1.

Wright, Jonathan V., and John Morgenthaler. *Natural Hormone Replacement: For Women Over 45.* Smart Publications, 1997.

Johnson, M., et al. "Hormone replacement risks drive natural alternative sales." *Drug Store News* Nov. 18, 2002; 33–34.

Legato, M. "Women's perception of their general health with special reference to their risk of coronary artery disease: Results of a national telephone survey." Columbia University Women's Health Center, *Journal of Women's Health* 1997; 6:2.

CHAPTER 19: A FINAL WORD

Thorton, K., DeFronzo, R., Sherwin, R. "Micronized estradiol and progesterone: Effects on carbohydrate metabolism in reproductive-age women." *Journal of the Society for Gynecologic Investigation* 1995; 2:4:643–652.

Moyer, M.P., Armstrong, A., Aust, J.B., et al. "Effects of gastrin, glutamine, and somatostatin on the in vitro growth of normal and malignant human gastric mucosal cells." *Archives of Surgery* 1986; 121:285–288.

Gerha, M., Walsh, B.W., Tawakol, A., et al. "Estradiol therapy combined with progesterone and a endothelium-dependent vasodilatation in postmenopausal women." *Circulation* Sept. 1998; 98:12:1158–1163.

Index